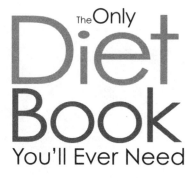

The Only
Diet
Book
You'll Ever Need

The Only Diet Book You'll Ever Need

The Secret to Eating Well, Losing Weight, and *Loving* Life

Cyndi Targosz

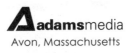

Avon, Massachusetts

Published by
Adams Media, an F+W Publications Company
57 Littlefield Street, Avon, MA 02322
www.adamsmedia.com

ISBN-10: 1-59869-439-1
ISBN-13: 978-1-59869-439-0

Printed in Canada.

J I H G F E D C B A

Library of Congress Cataloging-in-Publication Data
Targosz, Cynthia.
  The only diet book you'll ever need / Cyndi Targosz.
     p.   cm.
  Includes index.
  ISBN-13: 978-1-59869-439-0 (pbk.)
  ISBN-10: 1-59869-439-1 (pbk.)
  1. Weight loss. 2. Reducing diets. I. Title.
RM222.2.T316 2007
613.2'5—dc22   2007030951

This publication is designed to provide accurate and authoritative information with regard to the subject matter covered. It is sold with the understanding that the publisher is not engaged in rendering legal, accounting, or other
professional advice. If legal advice or other expert assistance is required, the
services of a competent professional person should be sought.
                    —From a *Declaration of Principles* jointly adopted by
                        a Committee of the American Bar Association and a
                                Committee of Publishers and Associations

Many of the designations used by manufacturers and sellers to distinguish
their product are claimed as trademarks. Where those designations appear
in this book and Adams Media was aware of a trademark claim, the designations have been printed with initial capital letters.

Contains materials adopted and abridged from *The Everything*® *Dieting
Book* by Sandra K. Nissenberg, M.S., R.D., Copyright © 2003 by F+W Publications, Inc.

This book is available at quantity discounts for bulk purchases.
For information, please call 1-800-289-0963.

Contents

Introduction

Pssst, let me whisper. . . . *I know you want to lose weight.* You've probably tried numerous times in the past and been unsuccessful. It may just be those stubborn last five pounds, or it could be the sixty you gained that are still expanding out of control. Perhaps it seems that nobody understands how depressed this is making you. You may even joke about the excess girth when in truth you are embarrassed by what seems to be total failure. Maybe you just want to look your best and are searching for information to be healthy. In any case don't worry! Your feelings are safe with me.

I care and sincerely want to help you help yourself. Escape within the realms of my diet program and I will share with you what I call my *Cyndi's Secrets*™. I've used these secrets to help numerous friends, family, and clients achieve their personal bests.

First of all, to lighten up you have to lighten up! This is going to be fun! I'll feed you the information you need to know, we'll have a few laughs, you'll run with the knowledge for success, and we'll move on. We'll discuss stuff like how to get motivated, what to eat, and how much to eat. I'll show you how you can take the new and proven dietary guidelines and make them your own. You can set realistic goals as I take you through the steps to achieve them. And, yes, you can get results that will last a lifetime.

With my personal secrets to a healthier lifestyle, *Cyndi's Secrets*™, you will gain much more than a just great body! Now let me shout it out—

eat well,
lose weight,

and most important,

love life!

1

Is Weight **Weighing** on Your Mind?— Lighten Up!

The Fat Stats

This journey shall begin with what I call "the Fat Stats." You know, those gloomy statistics that are so depressing they can drive any one of us to a doughnut shop for a pure panic pastry attack. I'm talking about those nasty numbers that make you want to throw your arms up and say, "why bother?" After all, it is estimated that almost 40 million Americans are obese—about one-third of all adults and one in five children. More than 50 percent of our entire population is considered overweight.

As a result of this high incidence, obesity is reported to contribute to at least 300,000 deaths in this country and hundreds of millions of dollars in health care costs each year. Before you grab that glazed confection, let's look at this scenario a little more closely. Being aware of the fat stats and putting my program into practice can help you change those figures—well, at least *your* figure. And that's the one that counts!

In the old days, being overweight and even obese was a sign of prosperity and wealth. The more prosperity and wealth we had, the better we ate and the more corpulent we looked. Perhaps that is the real reason why the fat king in the fairy tale, *The Emperor's New Clothes*, ran around naked. He probably really was showing off his extra girth to prove his gross worth. Who knew it was a PR stunt? What a catch! Today, we look at body weight in just the opposite way. The smarter we are, the richer we are, the more visible we are, the thinner we want to be. We feel that our weight reflects on us as a person. Excess weight makes us look as though we don't take care of ourselves. There is much we can discover from these very diverse attitudes.

The good news is that, finally, you are holding in your hands a diet plan that sorts it out. We shall explore this further in my program.

Cyndi's Secrets™

In the United States, more than 50 percent of women and more than 25 percent of men consider themselves on a diet!

First, it is imperative that we define the terms *overweight* and *obesity*. They are often used interchangeably in speech, but they are quite different in meaning. An overweight person is defined as one who carries extra weight in the form of muscles, bones, water, and fat. An overweight person could be a competitive athlete who may have increased muscle mass or a person with short stature who may have a large bone structure. On the other hand, an obese person has an excess of body fat only. His or her weight is found in extra fat stores throughout various parts of the body. Knowing this can help you understand where you really weigh in and how much you realistically need to lighten up!

Excess Weight—Risky Business

There are no two ways to look at excess weight—quite simply, it's risky business! Unless you are yearning for unhealthy drama in your life, there are plenty of good reasons to take off extra pounds. Just losing as few as ten or twenty pounds can do wonders to improve your overall health. Getting to know obesity risks and understanding your body shape can serve as tools to help you prevent disease as well as significantly improve your outlook on life. Oh, and did I forget to mention that you just might look hotter than before, which can rev up your self esteem tenfold? Hey, baby—toss those attitude shirts away. You don't need them. Newfound confidence after healthy weight loss is in the writing all over your face. And if excess weight is risky business, making these healthy improvements can be risky, too—you just might like the new you!

The Risks of Being Obese

Here are some of the risks of being obese:

- Being obese puts people at risk for some types of cancer, diabetes, heart disease, stroke, arthritis, gallbladder disease, and hypertension (high blood pressure)—some of which are leading causes of death in America today.
- Being obese adds stress to the body; extra weight makes your body work harder to function—it becomes harder to breathe, move, and keep the heart beating normally.
- Being obese causes depression; it is not uncommon to find many obese persons who are depressed about life in general.
- Being obese reduces your self-esteem.

- Being obese may cause discrimination; obese individuals can face discrimination at work, school, and in social situations, too.

Obesity as a Disease

People who carry excess weight are often ridiculed for putting it on and keeping it on. Until recently, obesity in a person was thought of as a sign of the person's lack of willpower. It was a stigma assigned to people who were thought to have no control over what and how much they ate. Although many people still have this prejudice, medical experts now categorize obesity as a disease, just like heart disease, diabetes, high blood pressure, and cancer. It's a disease that many people have no control over. It's time to exhibit some compassion, people!

Recent efforts by medical experts and the National Institutes of Health have labeled obesity as a disease—a disease that is caused in part by genetics, the environment, and psychological factors. It is known to lead to other chronic diseases, including heart disease, stroke, diabetes, gallbladder disease, arthritis, high blood pressure, and some forms of cancer. All of these chronic conditions can lead to illness and even premature death. I'm not just talking about adults. The number of overweight children and teens has risen more than 200 percent in the last decade. That's a scary stat! Obviously, not everyone needs to be as slim, as trim, and the size of a model. In fact, for many

Cyndi's Secrets™

Try carrying around a twelve-pound bowling ball for a day. Sound exhausting? That's extra stress on your heart and body, just like when you have too much body fat.

individuals who *do not* need to lose weight, weight loss offers no health benefits and can often be more harmful than helpful. However, for those who *do* need to lose the weight, losing even ten, twenty, or thirty pounds can bring on tremendous health benefits—decreasing blood pressure, reducing blood glucose levels, lowering cholesterol, increasing self esteem, and even bringing on a sense of accomplishment.

How Your Shape Affects Health Risk

Every person is shaped differently. Two people can be the same height and the same weight and yet be built in totally different ways. Your size, your shape, and how you work that body can raise or lower your risk of obesity. That means you can gain a lot from understanding your body type—I mean "lose" a lot! There is more than one way to study different body types. For our purposes we will bite into an apple- and pear-shape discussion.

Apple versus Pear. Where a person carries his excess weight is a determinant of overall health risk. Men or women who store fat around their stomach or middle portion of the body are at greater risk of complications than those who carry weight on their hips, thighs, or buttocks. This is largely because the fat that accumulates around the vital bodily organs is more critical than that which accumulates around the legs and thighs. Often compared to the shape of an apple or a pear, body shapes are important in assessing risk of obesity-related health concerns.

Waist-to-Hip Ratio. Are you an apple or a pear? Many of us instinctively already know from years of scrutinizing our bodies where we pack on excess pounds. However, using the waist-to-hip ratio formula can help you determine with more accuracy where your fat accumulates and help you to understand your body type better. Measure your waist at the narrowest spot. Then measure your hips at the widest spot. Divide the inches from the waist measurement by the inches of the hip measurement. For example, a person with a 38-inch waist and 40-inch hips would calculate her ratio like so: 38 divided by 40 = 0.95. A person with a 30-inch waist and 40-inch hips would calculate as 30 divided by 40 = 0.75. Women with ratios lower than 0.80 and

Live YOUR *Life*

Stop dwelling on your weight! Be proud that you have made the decision to alter your lifestyle. Often, that's the hardest step!

men with ratios lower than 1.0 are considered "pear-shaped." Women who have a ratio greater than 0.80 and men who have a ratio of greater than 1.0 are considered "apple-shaped." They are therefore at greater health risk due to their body shape and fat distribution.

Whether you are a pear or an apple shape, there are plenty of things you can do to look and feel your best. I always say that whether you are a pear or an apple, at least you can have a juicy life!

Why Are You Fat? The Blame Game

We've established the fact that adults and children are fatter than ever before but what about you? If you are overweight or obese you should ask yourself—why? It's very easy to point fingers when we don't feel very good about ourselves. Besides health-related issues, there are many other factors that can contribute to obesity in our society. Gadgets like the remote control, garage door openers, computers, and video games are just some of the contributing factors. People just don't have to move anymore to do what they need to do and get what they need to get. Kids are not as active as they used to be. Transportation is available everywhere. School physical education programs are limited in many schools. And the abundance of fast foods, convenience foods, and frequent snacks tends to cause additional weight gain. Poor eating habits in parents also lead to poor eating habits in children. These habits are passed on from generation to generation. As a result, children are more overweight than ever before. Their risk rises with obese parents, and even more so with obese siblings. To really understand these factors and understand why you may be overweight, let's explore.

What Causes Obesity?

This is simpler than most of us care to admit. The majority of people become obese from eating too much and/or not moving enough. If you consume more food than your body needs or use up less energy than your body takes in, then you are going to gain weight.

Heredity and Genetic Factors. Nowadays, it seems that everyone is blaming their weight gain on heredity and genetics. It is true that for a small number of individuals these factors could come into play. Genetic factors can result in endocrine problems as a result of an underactive thyroid. That means the metabolism slows down, which can contribute to weight gain. If you truly are dealing with serious genetic factors, my heart goes out to you. However, you can offset the hand of cards you were dealt by paying close attention to a healthier lifestyle and using the suggestions in my program.

On the flip side, many people may want to *believe* that their problem is genetic. This is most often the exception rather than the rule. It's not uncommon for obesity to run in families. However, it's most likely that a combination of genetics with lifestyle and eating habits is to blame.

Environmental Factors. A person's environment also can contribute to obesity. Take a look at your own surroundings. If you live and work in a place where everyone eats large meals and acts like a couch potato, it's likely that your habits will follow suit. And, of course, your overall size may be a factor in extra weight gain.

For example—I am petite with a small body mass due to my genetics. A small body mass means there should

Cyndi's Secrets™

Obesity runs in families not only because family members share the same genes, but also because they share the same lifestyle habits. More often than not, the fat is in our "jeans" because we put it there.

be less to feed. I confess though that there are times I want to wolf down the same if not bigger portion sizes that my larger and taller counterparts can. It doesn't seem fair, but it is what it is.

Being aware of these factors can help you conquer a potential or current weight problem. What we know about gaining weight is simple: What goes in must be balanced with what goes out. With my program, you will discover how to balance your food intake with your physical activity to maintain a healthy weight.

History of Habits

Eating habits result from a learned behavior that is practiced over and over again. These are often difficult to break because they have been repeated for years. Some examples of eating habits include drinking coffee every morning, having dessert after a meal, or having a dish of ice cream every night before you go to sleep.

People form habits from their infant years through childhood as they are taught by their parents, caregivers, and role models. You know, just like the family of four at the theater. The ones that march in one by one, each carrying a big buster bucket of buttered popcorn, 40-ounce soda, and candy, and are first in line for free refills. This becomes their norm. The types of foods, where these foods are eaten, snack choices, and exercise patterns are all habits formed early in life. Good habits are as easy to create as bad ones are, but if parents reinforce unhealthy habits—usually meaning that they practice these habits themselves—it is likely that these habits will be passed on to younger generations as well. Par-

Live YOUR *Life*

Discover your desirable weight and enjoy life while you reach for your goals. Let me help you create new, healthy eating patterns without starving. You can enjoy lots of yummy foods!

ents also serve as their children's role models to help them get on the path toward their own independent lifestyles. If good patterns are not taught early, they are difficult to pick up later. So if your parents taught you bad habits you might as well just blame them and forget about it! No—I'm just kidding you. Be proactive and use this valuable information to make positive choices.

Examining the Way You Live

First, begin by evaluating your lifestyle and food-style trends. Put a check mark in the appropriate column.

How's My Lifestyle?

	ALWAYS	OCCASIONALLY	NEVER
I eat regular meals and snacks daily.*	O	O	O
I eat breakfast every day.	O	O	O
I eat a variety of foods from each food group daily.**	O	O	O
I eat at least six grains or grain products daily.***	O	O	O
I eat at least three different vegetables each day.	O	O	O
I consume at least three varieties of fruit or juice each day.	O	O	O
I eat at least two servings of low-fat dairy products daily.	O	O	O
I eat lean beef, chicken, fish, eggs, or legumes twice daily.	O	O	O
I limit my intake of high-fat and high-sugar foods.	O	O	O
I choose many high-fiber foods each day.	O	O	O
I choose healthy, nutritious snack foods.	O	O	O
I drink at least six cups of water (or clear fluids) daily.	O	O	O
I accumulate at least thirty minutes of physical activity daily.	O	O	O
I get at least six to seven hours of sleep each night.	O	O	O
I limit alcoholic beverages to no more than one each day.	O	O	O
I try to eat out no more than three times each week.	O	O	O

*at least three meals and one to two snacks/day

**breads/cereals, fruits, vegetables, dairy, meat/protein

***choosing primarily whole grains

Now, look at your check marks. If you really are on top of your lifestyle, you will have checked off all answers in the "always" column. This is your aim. Here, this would mean you have a very healthy lifestyle and very good habits. If you have several marked off in the "always" column and several in the "occasionally" column, you're on your way to a better lifestyle. If, by chance, you marked any answers in the "never" column, you need to make some changes. I'm here to help you do just that.

Commit to Change—You Can

Don't close the book on me! There is a reason that you are here right now in this moment in time and we are connected. It's human nature to put off things we do not like to do—like studying for an exam, finishing a home improvement project, or starting to watch our weight. Rather than looking for an excuse, embrace this opportunity to make a positive change once and for all in your lifetime.

You picked up this book to help yourself accomplish a goal. Whether you want to educate yourself about dieting, change your eating style, or you just want to look and feel your best, I am here to help. Your first plan of action is to set some initial goals.

Setting Goals

Committing to change requires some serious goal setting. You have to have a strong purpose that drives you. Let's say your primary goal is to lose twenty pounds. And—heck!—why not try to keep it off? This can be your long-term goal.

But how do you get to that goal post with the fewest fumbles? You have to change your eating habits, exercise, shop for new fruits and vegetables, adjust your attitude, and lots of other good stuff. I won't overwhelm you right now. We can do it in baby steps. The point is—set goals!

Long-Term and Short-Term Goals

Success of any type is built on establishing long-term and short-term goals—goals that are realistic and challenging. Long-term goals help you imagine where you want to be a year from now. Short-term goals set your plans for the upcoming week or month. These are more realistic goals that are easily attainable. If you make these short-term goals weekly, one each week, you can bring on over fifty changes in one year. Or, if you prefer, try one each month and incorporate twelve in a year. And I'm talking about small changes. These short-term changes help you meet and accomplish the long-term goals.

Long-term goals should not be impossible to meet, but should be challenging like these:

- I want to get in good enough shape to run a marathon.
- I want to go on a two-day, 100-mile bike race.
- I want to wear a size ten by next summer.
- I want to win the lottery! (Hey—it could happen!)

Short-terms goals should be those that can be met without a great deal of effort. These short-term accomplishments help reinforce that changes can be made while motivating you to continue striving for success, like these:

- I will walk for fifteen minutes each day.
- I will reduce after dinner snacks to smaller, healthier choices.
- I will eat breakfast at least three mornings each week.
- I will put out a fruit basket each day with different varieties of fruit to try.
- I will cut down the amount of soft drinks I drink to one each day.
- I will buy a lottery ticket rather than a doughnut.

Your Own Personal Goals

Now it is time for you to set some initial goals for yourself. Having personal goals is exciting! Ask yourself the following questions:

- What do I want to accomplish in the next year?
- What do I want to accomplish in the next month to help meet this goal?
- What do I want to accomplish in the next week to help meet this goal?
- What do I want to accomplish today?

With your personal goals in place, let's get started. You have identified the need to lose some weight; your engine is revved up. You've set some initial goals for yourself, and you are ready for success. Forget failure! Let's rock and roll!

Please realize that I am here to help you make long-term lifestyle changes—changes that can last a lifetime. Keep in mind that attempts to lose weight should not be temporary. "Dieting" is not a temporary state. Losing and maintaining a healthy weight is something you should want to do for you, not for your mother, not for your spouse, and not for your best friend. Oh, who am I kidding? It's also okay to appreciate the second glances that are sure to come your way when friends and strangers see the new you. Just be sure that you do it for yourself first. This is a lifelong commitment that takes education, determination, and a desire to be as healthy as you can be—for *you!*

2 Understanding
Your Weight

The Bathroom Scale—
Buddy or a Bother?

The bathroom scale is the most common tool people use to help determine their body weight. Whether you consider it a friend or foe is a matter of debate. Who among us doesn't cringe when we step on the damn thing?

I almost passed out at the doctor's office once when I stepped on the monster and shuddered at a sudden ten-pound gain. I breathed a sigh of relief when I realized that my tote bag was still on my shoulder. Oops!

Let's face it—the scale is often taken too seriously and, of course, it is one of the most hated contraptions that we use on a regular basis. Over and over again, people continue to "torture" themselves by weighing in, while constantly complaining about the dreaded results. Can't we all just get along and meet half "weigh"?

How do you feel about your scale? Ask yourself:

- Do you weigh yourself first thing every morning and again at night?
- Do you weigh yourself more than three times each week even if away from home?
- Do you judge yourself by the numbers you see on the scale?
- Does your weight for the day determine your day's mood?
- Do you often dwell on the number you see?
- Do you swear or curse at the scale because the numbers disappoint you?
- Do you often insist on dropping a few pounds before you will buy yourself a new outfit?
- Do you constantly discuss your desire to lose weight?

If you answered yes to two or more of these questions, you are not alone, but you need to think more clearly about your relationship with your scale and particularly with your body weight. Too many of us define ourselves by a particular number and think less of ourselves if we don't meet our own expectations. Are you spending too much energy worrying about your weight? Whether or not you choose to use the bathroom scale on a regular basis, it still remains your most accessible tool for determining body weight.

Cyndi's Secrets™

The bathroom scale is great for charting body weight, but it doesn't consider bone structure, muscle mass, genetics, or other factors that contribute to weight. Use it as a friendly guideline. I've got a foothold on mine.

If and when you do use your scale, the following tips will yield the most accurate results:

Use the same scale. Different scales may present different results. Also be sure the scale sits on a "flat" floor, not carpeting.

Weigh yourself no more than one time each week. Select the same day, same time. Body weight can fluctuate. The best way to evaluate your body weight is to weigh yourself in the morning, preferably before you have eaten, and without clothing.

Stand straight in the middle of the scale. Your scale can record different numbers based on where and how you stand on it. You will get the best and most accurate readings by standing straight up and with your feet planted in the center.

Understand body changes. Menstrual cycles, sodium intake, and medications can all influence water retention and, therefore, water and body weight.

Healthy Body Weight Is Hot!

The "thin is in" mantra may still permeate part of our American culture but the big trend in America is finally moving in the direction of "healthy body weight." That's hot! Advertisers like Dove are using real women with real curves. Women with "junk in the trunk" are the new sex symbols in music videos, and there's even work for both plus-size and petite models. This is a major step forward from just a few years back. Nevertheless, too many Americans are still preoccupied with their body weight. More than half of women and more than one-third of men are dissatisfied with their shape, size, or body weight. And these obsessions are even higher among our younger population. In many cases, people see themselves as much worse off than others see them. How do you see yourself? What can we do about this?

Is Body Weight Constant Throughout Life?

There are many people who focus on a set body weight based on the chart found on the wall of the doctor's office or illustrated in a book. Some believe that this number is set in stone and that it should not vary throughout adult life. They think that their weight in their twenties should remain constant through their thirties, forties, and beyond. Focusing on a set number can be the first step in developing an obsession with body weight. Too many times, people dwell on what they weighed when they got married or before they had a child. (Isn't it funny how we can clearly remember these numbers?) This obsession can take over your life and can lead to problems with health, depression, and your overall well-being. I'm not saying you should let yourself go and become obese or overweight, but realize that our bodies do change as we age. Fear not—with my program you *can* look and feel your personal best at any given point in time.

Live YOUR *Life*

American society places way too much emphasis on body weight and size. Know who you are as a person, on the inside, rather than focusing solely on your outside appearance. In the meantime, aim for a healthier attitude. Instead of seeking to be thin, try to be your personal best. Remember—healthy body weight is *hot!*

Who Decides What's Ideal?

Once upon a time there was a group of insurance people, probably with potbellies, sitting around a table and—guess what? They created a measurement for determining an "ideal" weight for a person based on the height and weight ratios of insured persons with the greatest lifespan. Two charts were and still are generally used, one for those nineteen to thirty-four and another for those thirty-five and older. People looked up their height and age on these charts. The charts gave a range in which their weights should fall, with the midpoint being that person's "ideal."

Over the years, health researchers and nutrition professionals determined that the height/weight chart measurements were not as accurate as they could be and that these numbers did not take into account optimal body composition, including fat distribution. Many people swore by the numbers on the chart, but in fact these were not always the best measurement of our population as a whole. Next time you see the chart, check it out—because who can resist looking? Just remember to pause and smile and know from whence it came.

Determining a Healthy Weight

Your personal healthy body weight is a range for your particular body build that takes into account total fat, muscle, bone, and water for your size. This weight varies from person to person. Your ideal weight should be somewhere between being in an underweight status and an overweight status. In other words—not too fat, not too thin, but just right!

Healthy Weight versus Normal/Ideal Weight. Today, standards regarding weight have changed. Many health professionals prefer to use the term *healthy weight* rather than referring to one's "normal" or "ideal" weight. A *healthy* weight depends on a number of factors—age, gender, height, and frame or body size.

You may say "normal," I say "healthy," and others say "ideal." I really don't care which term works for you. Just work with me to help you get there.

Charts created recently are more accurate because they take into account total body composition: muscles, bone, fat, and all that good stuff. They provide ranges of numbers that are appropriate for individuals, rather than just a single number. Because no one person stays at the same weight for their entire life, and because bodies change over the years, no one weight is standard for a person during his or her entire life.

Live YOUR *Life*

Healthy weight should not be confused with your weight when you are your thinnest. It's okay to go through life with a mixture of both fat days and thin days. Our bodies change every day. What's important is to stay in your own individual hot healthy weight range.

Healthy Weight Ranges for Adults. One established chart helps individuals determine a "healthy weight range" for themselves. This chart takes a range of numbers into account, not just a single one, thereby allowing higher numbers for those people with larger body builds and greater amounts of muscle and bone. This chart is also useful for all adult age groups. While it is believed that people put on weight as they age, this weight gain should remain within the allowable range for height.

Body Composition—How Much Fat Do I Have?

Most people have used height/weight tables at one time or another. Health professionals often question their effectiveness but understand their basic purpose. These charts help primarily

Healthy Weight Range

HEIGHT*	WEIGHT**	HEIGHT*	WEIGHT**	HEIGHT*	WEIGHT**
4'10"	91–119	5'5"	114–150	6'0"	140–184
4'11"	94–124	5'6"	118–155	6'1"	144–189
5'0"	97–128	5'7"	121–160	6'2"	148–195
5'1"	101–132	5'8"	125–164	6'3"	152–200
5'2"	104–137	5'9"	129–169	6'4"	156–205
5'3"	107–141	5'10"	132–174	6'5"	160–211
5'4"	111–146	5'11"	136–179	6'6"	164–216

*in feet/inches (without shoes)
**in pounds (without clothes)

in determining whether a person falls into a healthy weight or not. Most of us like to look at these charts and see where we fall. Personally and professionally I take into account how much body fat a person has. This is a much more accurate measurement that can help you find where you are right now in relation to your healthy weight range.

Everybody needs a certain amount of fat in his or her body for energy sources, heat insulation, shock absorption, and various other vital functions. Women, for the most part, have greater fat stores than men. I know sometimes this doesn't seem fair but it is what it is. Nevertheless, determining how much body fat a person has is a difficult and somewhat costly process.

Cyndi's Secrets™

Men are considered obese when more than 25 percent of their weight is body fat; women are considered obese when more than 30 percent of their weight is body fat.

Weight Measurement Options

Several options are available, but in order to obtain accurate results, trained professionals and expensive equipment are often necessary. Let's take a look at some advanced options. Don't worry—I'll also provide some simple options that you can do in your own bathroom.

Underwater Weighing. One of the most effective ways to accurately measure lean muscle versus fat weight is through underwater (hydrostatic) weighing. Underwater weighing takes place by submerging a person in a tank of water about four feet deep as air is forced out of the person's lungs. After staying underwater for about six

> **Cyndi's Secrets™**
>
> Most women store fat in their hips, buttocks, thighs, and breasts, whereas men primarily store their weight in their abdomens, lower back, and chests.

to ten seconds, the person's weight is recorded. This method is based on the principles that people with greater muscle mass weigh more in water than those who do not and that fat floats in water. Therefore, more accurate measures of lean body mass can be recorded underwater. This process is repeated five to ten times. An average is then recorded and calculated according to a special formula to determine the percentage of total fat

WHAT YOU DON'T KNOW CAN MAKE YOU FAT	There is a theory that our bodies try to stay at a preset weight, called the "set point." The studies are inconclusive. However, if it exists it's probably a range, which means you can adjust your "set point" weight with exercise and a healthy diet. No excuses. Get the point?

weight. This method of determining body fat can be costly and is not widely available to most people. You know, I thought I witnessed underwater weighing once while visiting my uncle's waterfront home—but, to my surprise, it was his neighbor receiving baptism!

Bioelectrical Impedance Analysis. Another fat-measurement method, called "bioelectrical impedance analysis," is a relatively new and simple method. This process can determine overall body fat by providing a computerized calculation of lean weight, standard weight-range measurements, and percentage of body fat by delivering a harmless, low-voltage electrical current throughout the body.

This method produces an estimate of total body water and of lean muscle mass, which contains water. Water is an excellent conductor of electricity, while fat contains very little water and resists the electrical flow. The more body fat a person has, the more resistance there will be to the flow of the electrical current. From this measure of resistance, a percentage of body fat is determined. Again, although this method demonstrates accuracy, it is quite expensive and is not widely available for use by most people. I have done this one and it is really cool. It is, however, not a religious experience. No dunking needed.

Skinfold Measurement Testing. A simpler, more common measurement of fat in the body can be made through using skinfold calipers. These calipers are the most economical and the easiest tool to use to determine body fat composition. Trained individuals use this special tool to help determine the amount of body fat that lies just beneath the skin. This fat, which is called "subcutaneous fat," accounts for almost half of the body's overall fat supply. The process of testing involves taking a skinfold measurement of the thickness at various points of the body including the upper arm, upper back, lower back, abdomen, and thigh. The amount of subcutaneous fat found in these areas helps determine the total amount of fat that can be found throughout the body. This method is widely available at many health and fitness clubs and by physicians and dietitians, and it offers an effective means of proper measurement.

WHAT YOU DON'T KNOW CAN MAKE YOU FAT	Subcutaneous fat lies just beneath the skin and accounts for approximately half of all the fat in the body. Skinfold measurements of this fat taken on the thigh, upper arm, abdomen, and/or back helps to determine the total amount of fat found throughout the body.

Body Pinch Test. There are several other options for individuals to seek a quick and easy measurement of their own body fat. One is a simplified method of the skinfold caliper method, known as the body pinch test. You can easily do this yourself. Grasp the skin below the upper arm, halfway between the shoulder and elbow, and again at an inch below the waist. The skin, not the muscle, should be pinched with the thumb and forefinger. Take a measurement of the amount of skin grabbed. If the measurement is greater than an inch, an indication of an excess body fat can be made. The slogan "pinch an inch" was derived from this body pinch test. Yeah, I hate this one too. But if it makes you feel any better, even skinny models don't have a hard time finding an inch to pinch. Use it to get a quick assessment of excess fat. Perhaps this is something you can do when you have a date with your bathroom scale.

Waist Measurement. You can also assess your health risk by measuring your waist for the amount of excess fat around your middle, or around the vital organs in the body. A waist measurement of greater than thirty-five inches for women or forty inches for men indicates a risk to overall health status.

New Methods on the Horizon

New methods of determining body fat levels are being researched and developed. Some may require expensive equipment, while others can be found in products similar to the bathroom scale. Hopefully, individuals will have greater access to these testing methods.

Guidelines for Body Fat Determination

Each of these processes provides a person with his or her percentage of body fat. Guidelines established to determine healthy levels based on percentage of body fat are as follows:

YOU	NORMAL/HEALTHY	OVERWEIGHT	OBESE
Women	15 to 25 percent	25.1 to 29.9 percent	greater than 30 percent
Men	10 to 20 percent	20.1 to 24.9 percent	greater than 25 percent

Keep in mind that we all need some fat in our bodies to store energy, help with heat insulation, and perform other necessary functions. Women's bodies contain more fat than men's bodies do; women also have less muscle and bone than men.

Body Mass Index — Skinny Models versus You

In case you haven't heard, "skinny" models have been banned in Spain and in other areas of the world. Shocking as it may seem, this is setting a precedent for the whole fashion industry. Perhaps it's time to realize that a little meat on the bones is healthy. Regardless, I doubt that this will send celebrity anorexia headlines down a bulimic toilet. However, for the first time, the term *body mass index* (BMI) is being heard regularly in mainstream media and people are listening. Let's discover how this BMI business made popular by skinny models can help you achieve your goals.

What Is the Body Mass Index?

Developed in 1993 by the National Institute of Diabetes and Digestive and Kidney Disorders, the BMI uses a mathematical formula and chart designated to correlate body weight and height to overall body fat. Federal guidelines now use the BMI guidelines to define weight groups among Americans. Although BMI figures are not an appropriate weight evaluation tool for everyone, they are more accurate than the original height/weight tables. There are several simple ways in which you can determine your BMI. Following is a formula that you can use to calculate your own BMI.

Cyndi's Secrets™

Using BMI standards, only 41 percent of all Americans are classified at a healthy weight—39 percent of males and 44 percent of females.

Calculating Your Own BMI

Body mass index can be determined in a number of ways. Some ways are simpler than others. It is derived from the ratio of body weight in kilograms to height in meters squared. You can determine your own BMI by dividing your weight in pounds by the square of your height in inches, like so:

1. Divide your weight in pounds by 2.2 to get your weight in kilograms.
2. Divide your height in inches by 39.37 to get your height in meters.
3. Multiply the number you got in Step 2 (your height in meters) times itself.
4. Divide the number you got in Step 1 (your weight in kilograms) by the number you got in Step 3 (height in meters times height in meters).

Evaluating Your Results

Once you have calculated that infamous BMI number, check it out with the key found here. This information allows you to see how you fit into the standards established for a healthy weight.

It's interesting to note that the new skinny model BMI low limit number that caused such a ruckus in Spain is 18. That in itself is underweight according to this key. It is amazing to me how many in the fashion industry consider that fat. A BMI that is too low is not very attractive and certainly unhealthy.

Now it is up to you to step up to the plate. Not just for dinner but to achieve a healthy weight.

- Underweight status equals a BMI of 19 or below
- Healthy weight status equals a BMI of 19.1–24.9
- Overweight status equals a BMI of 25–29.9
- Obesity status equals a BMI of 30 or higher

Limitations of the Body Mass Index

Whatever your results may be, keep in mind that BMI figures can be limiting in several regards. For example if you are an individual with a really large percentage of muscle mass your measurements may indicate an overweight status. Primarily BMI charts are established for healthy, adult individuals, not children, pregnant women, athletes, or frail elderly persons. These charts are less indicative of weight issues in the younger population groups of children and teens. This information is primarily useful in determining personal health risks.

Each and every person who uses the BMI chart and figures needs to realize that these figures and numbers are only guidelines. These, as well as any height/weight chart you may find and compare to yourself, should not be your only indicator of a weight concern.

Live YOUR *Life*

If you are a model (male or female), or just envy them, do not let the pressure of being forced to have a low BMI bring you down. I know how cruel that world can be. Nothing is worth hurting your health for! Nowadays you can look good and succeed by being your personal best no matter what your size!

Meaning-Less Pounds, Sizes, and Numbers

I have been preaching about pounds, sizes, and numbers for years. In fact, I've done my share of obsessing over them, too. There have been times when I felt the pressure of preparing my body to be "camera ready" for a photo shoot or TV interview. It can be tough having your body scrutinized. As a celebrity image consultant I also talk to the "beautiful" people regularly. They can be more insecure than your average Joe Schmo. If there is anything I can share from these real life experiences, it is that pounds, sizes, and numbers are truly meaningless if you don't feel good about yourself. You must come to terms with the body that you were born with. Accept however tall or short you are and whatever size or shape or metabolism your genetics determine. Try to understand what you can change and what you cannot. Every person is different. Your opinion of yourself stems from how you accept *you*.

If you have concerns regarding body weight, I encourage you to talk to a health professional. Please do not put yourself down for not falling into a certain number or size that may be unrealistic. A health care professional or health care team can set you in the direction of a healthier lifestyle. Living healthy should be fun and feel good. Get more help if you need it.

We've talked a lot about testing our weight. Try to remember that an assessment of a person's weight is just that: an assessment. Numbers help in determining where you are at any given time so you can set goals. However, weight is only one measurement of health. A thin person may not always be healthier than an overweight person. Many factors contribute to your overall health. You can appear fit on the outside, but are you fit within? As we progress through these pages, I will provide more information on ways for you to build a healthy lifestyle through the foods and activities you choose. Forget about trying to be thin. Becoming healthier should be your main focus. It's a positive change you really can make that should be fun and make you feel great!

3

Chocolate, Chips, & Ice Cream—
Why Choose These?

Tummy Talk—
What Your Cravings Tell You

Now it's time for some tummy talk, straight from the gut. I'm sure you have heard your tummy grumbling, "give me chocolate, pizza, ice cream," or whatever you are craving. Your cravings and what you eat say a lot about your character, your personality, and where you are from. They can reflect family history, culture, and religious background, economic status, how you feel, where you go, and what you do socially.

Ethnic Influences

Eating and choosing foods is no longer just about nutrition and feeding your body what it needs and what tastes good. Your ethnic background is often apparent in the foods you eat. Food practices are different from culture to culture and from generation to generation. Whether your background is European or African, Asian or Latin American, these influences contribute to the foods you eat and bring into your home. I'm 100 percent Polish, and craving kielbasa (Polish sausage) is definitely tied to warm, fuzzy memories of my beautiful mom preparing dinner for dad and us eight kids. Jeez— I can actually smell it as I'm writing this. There are many foods we crave because of ethnic influences.

Religious Influences

Religious groups like Muslims, Seventh-Day Adventists, and Jews also can influence individual food and beverage dietary practices. Muslims are known to fast at certain times during the calendar year; many Seventh-Day Adventists follow strict vegetarian practices and avoid alcohol, coffee, and tea; and some Jews observe kosher dietary laws. People of these, and other, backgrounds may be very strict or somewhat lenient with their followings. I'm Catholic and hardly ever eat meat. It's funny but the only time I really crave it is during our religious season of Lent when we are supposed to fast. It figures!

Regional Influences

America has its own collection of favorite flavors. Each region is known for its distinct types of foods. The wide number of ethnic heritages, national resources, and diverse types of people found throughout these regions largely contributes to these preferences.

The South originated foods like hush puppies and cheese grits. The Southwest is known for its Mexican American foods. The Northeast is famous for its supply of seafood and fresh fish, and the West Coast, with its warm weather and trendy lifestyle, is where you can often find fresh foods and Asian/Pacific foods.

Social Influences

Our social existence is probably one of the biggest contributors to what we eat. The people you live with, work with, and socialize with have a great deal of influence over your diet. Friends, peers, and colleagues may try to make your food choices for you during a coffee break or at lunch. "Let's grab a latte and doughnut," or "How about a burger and fries for lunch today?" Uh oh! There goes that tummy again, talking to you through your cravings. Sometimes your brain has to tell it to shush. If you are a teenager it's common to eat like your friends and peers. They might choose foods like pizza, French fries, hot dogs, shakes, and soft drinks. Your tummy may tell you to choose these foods because they look good and everyone else is eating them. On the other hand your peers might choose to starve themselves in order to "trim down." Don't let that unhealthy tummy talk take you to a negative place.

Live YOUR *Life*

Frequent television watchers are more likely to "feel" fatter than their non-watching counterparts, often due to the images that models and celebrities portray. Snacking during commercials doesn't help either.

People eat for reasons other than hunger. It could be because it's time to eat, because others are eating, or even because the food is there—it looks good and smells good. People are often labeled by the type of eater they are—a slow eater, fast eater, or a person who never eats sweets. Some people respond to environmental cues, such as an event or situation that triggers eating. The sight, smell, or familiar taste of a food can be a cue to stimulate eating. Social events, like parties, mealtimes, and watching television or going to the movies all serve as eating triggers, too.

Family Influences

Your family's eating and purchasing decisions provide the greatest input into your current food habits. How your parents fed you—what foods were brought into the home, how you celebrated special occasions, and so on—led to the way that you eat. These environmental factors probably have the largest impact on your overall food decisions today.

Modern families are different and more widely diverse than ever before. We see many more single-parent households, many homes with two working parents, and various non-family individuals living together. Busy schedules also reflect on eating decisions. The majority of our meals are no longer prepared from scratch and over a stove. Many nights go by without a hot meal being prepared in the home at all. The frequency of res-taurant dining, fast food, and convenience dinners has eclipsed more traditional meals. Of course, who could live without our friend the microwave? It has now become the favored kitchen appliance—heat it up in minutes. Activities and family sched-ules now take priority over home-cooked meals.

> **Cyndi's Secrets™**
>
> A craving is a strong desire to eat a par-ticular food. Women often desire choco-late as hormone levels change. Satisfy the urge with a single decadent chocolate miniature. Savor it! Of course, do not eat the entire box.

Cravings

Cravings also lead a person to eat. A craving is defined as a strong desire to eat a particular food. That is when your tummy is talking extra loud to you. It can scream, "feed me!" any time of the day or night. Hormones can really pump up the volume of tummy chatter, particularly in women, as observed during pregnancy and episodes of premenstrual syndrome. Dieters are also known to have frequent food cravings primarily because of the intense desire to eat too many so-called forbidden foods. You can calm the chatter by selecting healthier choices and just a "few" of those forbidden favorites.

Emotions

He dumped me! She fired me! I broke a nail! Well, better bring out the ice cream, pizza, chocolate, or beer. Unfortunately, it is way too easy to use food in more ways than to just meet hunger and nourish the body. Many people express their emotions, like love or sorrow, with food. Food tends to make some people feel better. That's why emotional food cravings are often called, "mommy food." This misuse of food acts as a false nurturing comfort. It fills an emotional void (as in the case of depression or loneliness).

Mixed Media Messages—Yikes!

Television, magazine, and newspaper ads are often a big factor in our purchasing and eating decisions. Coupons, store displays, tasting stations, and placement of a product on the grocery store shelf also encourage buyers to purchase it. The Internet is swarming with pop-ups. Nowadays you can't even watch a movie or a TV show without seeing an actor walk by eating or holding some edible item. Of course, the name brand is conveniently visible and on the screen just long enough to stick in your mind. Companies pay huge bucks for this subliminal product placement. They are determined to influence your decisions in any way possible and through every media outlet. The more you see and read about a new product, the more likely you will be to try it. This is not entirely bad. It is up to you to take responsibility and be a savvy consumer.

WHAT YOU
DON'T KNOW
CAN MAKE
YOU FAT

More than half of all food-related commercial advertisements are geared toward foods high in calories, fat, sugar, or salt.

Media madness is not going away any time soon. Its effect on eating behaviors is enormous and can be both good and bad. Not only are some foods advertised as the healthiest and newest variety available, but other "not-so-healthy" choices frequently pop up, too. The media also overvalues beauty as exemplified in slim and trim bodies. Many celebrities and models present these products to us. If they are a healthy weight it is only natural to appreciate their size and shape and become seduced to buy their product. I'm pleased that a few more companies are using real-size people, but that doesn't guarantee a healthy product. I've also noticed a disturbing psychological trend in some advertising. We are seeing healthy weight individuals in some ads portrayed as if they are heavy. For example I recently watched a popular cereal commercial where a very attractive woman was featured who had a healthy weight. She looked in the mirror at her body with disdain desperately hoping to lose weight. The cereal was, of course, her answer to losing pounds she didn't need to lose. I was appalled by this kind of consumer mind game. Watching this nonsense could surely make a healthy woman think she was "fat" by this media standard.

Commercials like these air everyday on television. In fact, you are bombarded by positive and negative influences all the time. So the next time you see these influences coming on, stop and try to make a decision for yourself. Is that what you really want to eat, or are you just trying to "fit in" with others? I feel strongly about taking responsibility. In order to move forward, ask yourself the following questions:

- Do you often agree to eat something just to go along with the crowd?
- Do others often make food decisions for you?
- Do you often buy something just because of an advertisement or television commercial, even if you know it's not the best choice?
- Do you tend to join friends for a meal, even if you don't care for the restaurant, just to be part of the group?
- Do you order foods you know your friends will like, just to have them like you better?

If you answered yes to two or more of these questions, then you need to become more aware of who is in control of your food decisions. Becoming aware of the influences that surround you is just one way you can begin to control your food intake and your overall health as well.

Life Sucks, So Pig Out—Not!

Experts have now defined hunger in terms of physical hunger and emotional hunger. Physical hunger is defined as the point at which the body informs you of the need for food, as in a growling stomach. In contrast, emotional hunger is when a person eats to satisfy an emotional response, like a reaction to anxiety, loneliness, or stress. You know that visit to the freezer whenever anything goes wrong? Let's face it—we all become emotionally upset at one time or another. It's a very human quality. However, when some people let their emotions get out of control they can—and often do—turn to eating out of control. Over time, this emotional and out-of-control hunger can cause eating problems. This can lead to food-related disorders like obesity and compulsive eating.

Food can bring on and satisfy many emotions—joy, excitement, anxiety, and even stress. People develop many emotional responses to food. Here are a few examples:

- As a child were you ever given a treat to stop crying, or promised an ice cream cone if you were good?
- Did your parents ever threaten to take away your dessert if you didn't eat your meal?
- Does boredom or loneliness ever send you in search of a snack in the refrigerator?
- Do you find yourself grabbing a cookie just after you've gotten upset or dishing out ice cream just because you are bored?
- Do you make popcorn just because you are going to watch a movie?
- Do you reach for certain foods referred to as "comfort foods," like macaroni and cheese, meat loaf, or mashed potatoes, because they bring you comfort?

So did you find some familiar behaviors within yourself? You can now begin to understand why you react to food the way you do! It seems simple now that you think about it this way, doesn't it?

If you use food to relieve stress, anxiety, boredom, or loneliness, then you are sure to have negative consequences. Using it as a reward or punishment is just as bad. Doing so gives food the power to control you and your emotional responses. Be careful not to send a message that food is the answer to all your problems. Don't let food rule your life. Rather, you rule!

Discovering Your Eating Pattern

Now it's time to nail down your eating patterns. Do you find that environmental cues lead you to eat more frequently or that you have intense cravings for certain foods? Do you consider yourself a slow eater, a fast eater, an evening eater, a grazer, a member of the clean-the-plate club, or do you have your own label for the type of eater you are? Do you think you eat frequently as a result of stress or as a response to an argument with your boss or spouse? Let's explore why and when you eat. Answer these questions:

Live YOUR *Life*

Identify common behaviors, like eating in front of the TV or snacking in the car, along with emotions like stress, anxiety, or frustration, that may trigger overeating. Use this information to stop.

- Do I eat even if I am not hungry?
- Do I eat just because others I am with are eating?
- Do I often eat so fast that I don't enjoy my food or know what I am eating?
- If something upsets me or causes me stress, do I seek out something to eat?

- Do I find myself looking for food when I am lonely or depressed?
- Do I often skip breakfast and lunch but make up for it later in the day?
- Do I clean my plate at every meal because I do not like waste?
- Do I pick food off of my children's plates when they don't finish it?

If you said yes to any one of these, fess up! You are using food to do more than to fill a need for hunger. Each and every one of us can be guilty of this behavior. We just need to be aware of the cues that cause us to eat and control them appropriately.

Do I Eat Too Fast?

If you are a fast eater, it is time to consider holding your horses. There is much to be learned from your slow counterparts. Eating fast can cause obesity. It can cause digestive problems. On top of that, when you eat too fast you may not taste or enjoy your food as much as you could. By eating food too fast, you might eat more than you really want to or definitely more than you might need. And if you are really in a hurry you may not even know what you just ate. Now that's a waste of calories!

It takes about twenty minutes from the time you begin eating to the time your stomach signals your brain that you might have had enough. If you continue to eat too quickly, it is possible to overfill your stomach. That can cause possible indigestion and discomfort. As a result, problems such as constipation, heartburn, or diarrhea may occur.

If you are a fast eater, don't deny yourself the opportunity to really enjoy your food. We all need to learn to sit back, relax, and take notes from those slow eaters. You'll find yourself feeling full, feeling better, and maybe even having some leftovers for another meal. That's the ticket— the meal ticket!

Cyndi's Secrets™

Eat slowly. It takes fifteen to twenty minutes for your stomach to signal your brain that it is full. Try soup, spicy foods, shellfish, or artichokes—they take longer to eat.

Am I a Grazer?

A *grazer* may seem somewhat sheepish but it is actually a term used for people who like to eat a lot of mini meals during the day. This often works well if you have a busy lifestyle. For a long time this was thought to be unhealthy. Current guidelines and most experts agree that eating five or six mini meals a day can be as healthy as eating three. We now look at the total diet for a day and even several days. Whether you eat three meals a day or many mini meals matters not. The key is to make smart food choices and lead an active lifestyle. Nibbling on potato chips every time you check your e-mail does not constitute a mini meal. Don't worry—I'll give you lots of tips to make smart food choices and how to keep active later in this program.

Do I Starve All Day and Eat All Night?

Do you ever find yourself saying, "I don't eat that much, so why am I so fat?" It's possible that you could be what I call "starving fat." It's a term I've given to people who skip breakfast, and sometimes lunch, and then scarf down everything in sight at dinner and during the evening. This is not a good eating pattern because you end up eating ten times more than is required in order to satisfy your hunger. When the body gets no food or fuel throughout the day, it begins to run down. At the point of physical hunger, almost anything and everything will look appetizing. Food will likely be consumed in more-than-adequate amounts. The body cannot use food as efficiently when it's fed this way. On top of it, most people wake up the next morning feeling fat again and the vicious cycle starts over.

Cyndi's Secrets™

People who skip meals generally have a slower metabolism than those who do not because depriving the body of food causes its metabolism to slow down. So don't skip any meals!

Do I Belong to the Clean-the-Plate Club?

Years ago, many parents, including mine, would say, "clean your plate." So I washed the dishes! Just kidding. Actually, we were told that kids all over the world were starving and that we shouldn't leave food on our plates. We were also told that food costs money, so we shouldn't throw it out. You may have heard these comments too. If they have stuck with you into adulthood it's possible that, subconsciously, you might to this day clean your plate because you want to be "good." Get over it. This can lead to problems with many individuals, because these plates may contain much more than you need to eat at one sitting. Especially with the huge portions available today.

It's not uncommon for parents with this kind of conditioning to also feel the need to clean their child's plate. Adults can learn a lot from young children: When they feel full, they walk away—often leaving food on their plates. Parents, in turn, need to walk away from this food too. There's no need to finish it off just to avoid throwing it out. Either learn to dish up smaller portions, or put it away for another time. What's the better choice—going to waste or going to waist?

Stop Overeating—Cyndi's Top Tips

Overeating is the act of stuffing yourself. It's often done at a holiday meal or a weekend splurge. Everybody pigs out once in a while, but be careful not to let this be a regular occurrence because if you do you are sure to pack on excess weight. Overeating is different from binge eating—when a person regularly, uncontrollably eats huge amounts of food in a short amount of time. That is a disorder that requires medical attention. To avoid the temptation to overeat, follow my top tips:

- *Chew your food.* Taking your time to savor every morsel can help you consume fewer calories. Chomping too fast just makes it easier to shovel it in. Relax and enjoy the moment.
- *Don't eat when you are stressed or bored.* If you are having a fight with your significant other, grab a jump rope rather than a jumbo order of fries.
- *Be aware of seasonal sneaky treats.* "Oh, its fall—better eat all those pumpkin chocolates since they are only out once a year." Or "Oh, it's summer—a few hot dogs and beers are in order." Get the picture?
- *Keep a food diary or journal.* By constantly evaluating your eating habits you can achieve weight management bliss for life.
- *Do a diet disappearing act.* Out of sight and out of mind. Don't make it a habit of keeping unhealthy food choices near you. If they disappear from your cupboard, you won't be tempted.

- *Don't skip meals.* Starving yourself only results in overeating later.
- *Focus on the "food."* When it is time to eat, focus on the food—and, of course, your company if you are not dining alone. Turn off the TV and computer and put down the phone. These distractions can cause you to eat too much.

Dear Diet Diary

Starting a diet diary is your first step in tackling some of the food-related behaviors that exist. Here you need to log the times you eat, your mood, hunger level, all of the foods eaten, and how much of each food you eat. This diary is just a sample of the type that may help you. I know! I know! Some people don't like to keep a journal. The thing is that as you learn more about what and how you should be eating, you can put it all together to help conquer your problems once and for all. So at least give it a shot. If a conventional notebook doesn't work you can always take notes by logging onto your computer. You could start a blog and share with others. Or you could just use your Palm Pilot, PDA device, or Blackberry to record what you eat. Even write it down on the calendar in your kitchen! It doesn't have to be the next best-seller, or even well written, for that matter.

Live YOUR *Life*

Do something other than eat! Take a warm bath, join a book club, make a fitness date, schedule a massage, or go to the movies. I find that brushing my teeth feels so good that I don't want to destroy the fresh taste in my mouth by having leftover spaghetti and ending up with garlic breath. It serves as a signal to stop eating.

In the pages of your diary, **time** refers to the time at which you eat. **Mood** is how you feel. Are you happy, sad, frustrated, stressed, or nervous? These moods can all affect your eating decisions. **Hunger level** refers to how hungry you are. Rate yourself from 1 to 5, 1 not being physically hungry at all and 5 being famished. **Food eaten** is the food you selected and ate. Be specific. **How much** indicates the portion size of the food you have selected. Again, be specific.

Sample Diet Diary

DAY 1				
TIME	MOOD	HUNGER LEVEL	FOOD EATEN	HOW MUCH

DAY 2				
TIME	MOOD	HUNGER LEVEL	FOOD EATEN	HOW MUCH

DAY 3				
TIME	MOOD	HUNGER LEVEL	FOOD EATEN	HOW MUCH

Now let's set a plan to make some changes. Remember, small changes can add up to big results.

- This week I will try to . . .
- This month I will try to . . .

Determining why and what you eat is the key to understanding and managing changes in your overall lifestyle. Just becoming aware of your behaviors can be the first major step in the right direction.

Start by using a diet diary for at least three to five days. Review your diary, or seek a professional to do so, and determine your problem areas and problem times during the day. Now is the perfect time to set some goals, short-term, to get yourself started and motivated. Take it one day at a time. As you begin to see positive results, you will likely feel better about yourself and what you can accomplish. Remember, you are doing this for you. Keep focused and keep motivated.

4

Dieting in **America**—
The Love/Hate Affair

A Fat Cat Industry

Hundreds of diets are created and shared with us every year. We spend billions of dollars keeping the weight-loss industry alive. And the fat cats who run these major corporations are not slim when it comes to offering consumers diets, gimmicks, beverages, powders, pills, equipment, and more. We find these every month in women's magazines, hear about them from friends, and see celebrities promoting their new "diet" books and products through commercial advertisements and infomercials. Not all of these are bad but be a selective consumer. Many diets claim to take off those extra pounds painlessly and effectively. Trends come and go, promising fast and easy results. I can see how you might get confused by everything out there, but don't worry, I've sorted through the junk for you. Finally you can get the results you desire (as long as they are realistic) with the sound, direct, and to-the-point information I provide in this program.

Weight-Loss Red Flags

We live in a world that has recently seen tremendous scientific and technological advances. With all this progress you may wonder why they haven't invented a pill you could pop that would allow you to eat all the goodies you wanted and still look spectacular. Unfortunately that magic potion has not been invented. Losing weight is just one of those things in life that cannot be accomplished through a quick process. It takes some discipline. (Which isn't a bad lesson to learn anyway!) As much as you may want to believe grandiose claims, an immediate red flag should go up if you see promotions like these:

> ### *Live* YOUR *Life*
>
> Anyone can make a claim about losing weight, sell a diet, or promote a weight-loss product. Beware of fraudulent moneymaking schemes.

- Miracle results
- Breakthrough
- New discovery
- Quick weight loss
- Magic pill, magic formula, or magical cure
- Secret formula

Not all products are bad if they use promotional terms. Most companies would not stay in business without some emotional form of advertising. However, be savvy and look beyond the packaging. It's your responsibility. Don't be sucked in by those fabulous success stories and promises like "drop ten pounds in a week," "shrink your stomach," and those remarkable before and after pictures. Are these really the same person? Why wouldn't you be intrigued? It sounds so good. But that may be just it—too good to be true.

Fad Dieting—Fact versus Fiction

I have to tell you straight up—losing weight the healthy way is not without its share of obstacles. But it can be fun and you can feel great for life. It requires much planning, insight, motivation, and of course a sense of humor. Fad dieting, on the other hand, is just that—a fad. Fad diets are trendy. They do not stay around for any length of time. They also can be risky and dangerous, and they rarely provide long-term, effective results. Most people gain their weight back and even add on more.

Your Desire to Lose—Quickly and Painlessly

Is it really so important that this weight come off today and now? Let's begin by looking at why you are desperate to lose:

- Are you so obsessed with the idea of losing weight that you would sacrifice your overall health?
- Do you often compare your size to that of another person?
- Do you think being obese makes you lazy, sloppy, and undisciplined?
- Do you believe that losing weight will make you well liked and popular among your friends?
- Do you insist on crash dieting before a big social gathering?

Responding positively to any of these questions puts you in the category for possibly being obsessed with your weight.

Trying Anything and Everything

Are you the type of person that wants to knock off those pounds really badly, so badly that you'll do anything to get them off? Perhaps you are willing to try any diet, weight-loss drink, and concoction available. You may even seek and follow advice from others. You know—the incredible diet you got from the waitress who heard about great results that her astrologist got from his sister who heard about a new diet from her masseuse who lost thirty pounds in a week. These "credible"—or, more directly, *not* credible—experts are the ones that too many people follow. You have to stop and think about what this non-authority advice could be doing to your body.

Many of these diets work initially and, yes, a few pounds come off. Who wouldn't get excited? However, the weight usually returns. Before you know it you are back to square one. This vicious cycle begins again and again. Sometimes you can be even worse off than when you started. Read on before you spin out of control.

Live YOUR *Life*

Many people resort to fad fasting diets. They believe this will "clean out" their system of toxic wastes. Instead, these diets produce body chemicals called "ketones" that burden the kidneys and can be harmful for health. They also cause fatigue, dizziness, and less energy.

Why the Hype?

Bad fad diets are categorized as those that promote quick weight loss. Usually they don't work, offer unrealistic promises, are restrictive, and can lead to health and related problems. Following are some common denominators that can be found in bad fad diets. Use this information to help you avoid frustration and possibly a feeling of failure.

- These diets are usually well below caloric recommendations, though not advertised as such.

- These diets are deficient in many nutrients, including carbohydrates and fiber, and many vitamins and minerals.
- These diets are well out of balance of dietary recommendations, requiring too many proteins and fats and too few carbohydrates or too many carbohydrates and too little protein and fat.
- These diets cause initial weight loss from body fluids, thus giving dieters a sense of accomplishment, when in fact the weight will soon return, and accomplishments will turn into failures.
- These diets do not promote portion size. They do not teach consumers how to eat in moderation.
- Many recommend that dieters follow suggested eating plans for extended periods of time.
- Often these diets discourage long-term compliance, knowing how harmful they may be if followed for extended periods of time.

| WHAT YOU DON'T KNOW CAN MAKE YOU FAT | Portion size is rarely addressed in a fad diet. The focus is primarily on eliminating an entire food category rather than just eating less of it. This can cause you to overestimate the amount of food you should eat and skip essential nutrients. |

The initial thought of a quick fad diet is encouraging to many people—just lose a quick five to ten pounds. However, the long-term consequences are much greater. Bad fad diets just don't work. Don't start a habit of being drawn in to these programs. You will just set yourself up for disappointment and a feeling of failure. Gradual changes that require long-term modifications to your eating patterns and lifestyle make more sense. If you are really willing to try anything to lose the weight, do it the right way.

The Mystery "Magic" Medications

Weight-loss medications have become very popular in our country. This may seem like the newest trend in weight loss but people have been taking some form of medication or concoction for eons in hopes of adjusting their weight. From the formula the local witch doctor may have whipped up to the medications offered today, the "magic cure" has unfortunately thrived. Some forty to fifty years ago doctors used to give out "diet pills." These primarily contained amphetamines, were highly addictive, and led to adverse effects on the heart and nervous system. Thankfully these compounds are no longer recommended for use in obesity treatment.

Other medications are easily purchased over the counter at the drugstore and are mostly known to decrease the appetite. These may work with obese people at increased risk for serious medical problems but

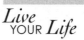

Live YOUR Life

Not all doctors are perfect. Just because the FDA regulates how a medication can be advertised or promoted doesn't mean your doctor properly pre-scribes it. Talk to more than one physician and do some research your-self if meds are in your future.

should not be used strictly for cosmetic reasons and certainly not without a physician's approval. Herbs, over-the-counter medications, and prescription medications are all drugs with potential side effects. Some are tested for their safety, but long-term studies take time. Testing each and every one of them is not possible. Always be cautious of any product that you take and be aware of possible health consequences that may result.

Common Side Effects
Common side effects of weight-loss medications may include:

- Irregular heartbeat
- High blood pressure
- Weakness/fainting/dizziness
- Anxiety
- Gallstones
- Headaches
- Anemia/low iron levels

- Seizures
- Nausea
- Heart attack/stroke
- High cholesterol
- Fatigue/tiredness
- Death

Recent Medication Developments
In recent years, various medications have been released to the public to help lose extreme amounts of weight. These products were promoted as a new type of appetite suppressant. Millions of prescriptions were written. The side effects were so horrible that they had to rightfully be removed from the market. To this day we often hear and see news alert stories splashed across the screen about some weight-loss product gone badly. But consumers still want the "magic" and voilà—guess what? There are countless new prescriptions, over-the-counter, and herbal remedies available. My best advice is: "buyer beware!"

WHAT YOU DON'T KNOW CAN MAKE YOU FAT | Diet drugs and medications are not intended for overweight and marginally obese people. The harmful effects of long-term use of these drugs and medications can outweigh the health benefits of losing weight.

Although people are more skeptical of product safety, they are still lining up to try the latest medication in hopes of dropping those extra, unnecessary pounds. Products like appetite suppressants, which are used to decrease appetite and increase satiety (the feeling of fullness), and products used to block absorption of fat and even starches can be found in abundance. Even if you find a good product that is sanctioned by your physician or health care provider, none of these products is marketed to work on its own. They usually recommend making lifestyle changes. This is often ignored like the legal gobbledygook at the end of a car commercial. People forget that, along with taking these "pills," there's no escaping the importance of decreasing total food intake and increasing activity levels.

At first, prescription medications were promoted to the severely obese. Even with their so-called side effects, these medications were believed by experts to be less of a health risk than being seriously obese. It was only a matter of time before more prescriptions were being written strictly for cosmetic reasons. Many of these people were less than severely obese. Today these medications are commonly abused. People need to realize that these drugs are powerful and can be harmful if not used properly.

Cyndi's Secrets™

Appetite suppressing medications can be harmful and should be used only by patients who are at increased risk of medical problems because of obesity and not for cosmetic reasons to lose weight. They should be used only under a doctor's supervision.

With use of these medications, pounds will be lost. But pounds will stay off only as long as the plan is continued. Once medications stop and old lifestyle habits return, pounds are regained. Medications are only a temporary solution.

Weight-Loss Medication Schemes

Beware of the following weight-loss medications and products. The Food and Drug Administration has banned many of them.

- *"Fat burners"*—These products include such ingredients as alcohol, caffeine, dextrose, and guar gum and claim to dissolve excess fat.
- *"Diet patches"*—These are promoted as a means to dispatch medication through a patch placed on the skin.
- *"Fat blockers"*—These promote the blockage of fat absorption.
- *"Starch blockers"*—These promote the blockage of starch absorption.
- *"Bulk fillers"*—Excess fiber in these fills the stomach and absorbs fluids, but can obstruct the digestive tract.
- *"Magnet-type" pills*—These are promoted as a way to flush out the body.

Herbal Remedies

Herbal remedies for general health are not all bad. I get excited by their potential and the thought of more research. However, when it comes to weight loss, many of these so-called natural products can be downright dangerous. They are available through health food stores, mall kiosks, Internet sites, weight-loss clinics, individual distributors, and drug stores. The Food and Drug Administration warns consumers about the harmful use of many of these products, as their safety and effectiveness have not been tested.

Many herbal products contain an amphetamine-like compound with potentially harmful stimulant effects on the heart and central nervous system. Some of these products act as diuretics (substances that increase urine production), thus causing water weight loss. Others are promoted to increase metabolism and decrease appetite. Products like these often can lead to undesirable side effects like insomnia, irregular heartbeats, tremors, headaches, irritability, and high blood pressure. There are still other products that offer the benefit of helping consumers feel satiated or full. These products tend to absorb fluids in the body, making a person feel fuller, but in reality they have little weight-loss benefit.

Weight-Loss Effects from Hot and Spicy Foods

Hot and spicy foods often are promoted as foods that can help increase your metabolism (the rate at which calories are burned). Reports indicate that these foods do not increase your metabolism, but may just increase your desire to consume liquids because of their hot, spicy flavors.

Going to Extremes: Surgery

With all the makeover shows on TV, you may be considering surgery as an extreme weight-loss option. Following are some available procedures.

Gastric Bypass Surgery: Shortens the intestines and makes the stomach smaller to facilitate weight loss. Although this can help some to lose weight, don't even bat an eyelash if you are not at least 100 or more pounds overweight. The side effects can be dangerous.

Adjustable Gastric Banding: This approach changes the stomach's capacity and emptying time to result in weight loss. There are many side effects.

Liposuction: A surgery that removes fat tissues from the body. This is a short-term solution. If eating and exercise patterns remain the same, the weight will be back.

If you are considering surgery, please understand that these options carry many health risks. Do your research. When all is said and done, perhaps the best extreme makeover you may need is to finally take extreme care of yourself and your own diet and exercise.

Free to Eat Really Well

I promised you a diet that really works. So what does that really mean? Today most people think "diet" is a painfully restricted eating program. It conjures up thoughts of starvation and gestapo rules of "You will eat this," and "You can't eat that!"

The definition of diet actually is "manner of living." Originally it was meant to encompass an entire approach to eating and daily activities. It's time to reclaim the original meaning and feel free to eat really well and enjoy a full, active life. I'm often amazed at how many people are shocked when I exuberantly proclaim, "I love to eat!" As you become more knowledgeable with my program you can make good food choices, too. Only 5 to 10 percent of people who use a restrictive diet keep the weight off for more than five years. Most of the weight is regained within a year.

None of the programs or products discussed in this chapter is the perfect diet solution. You need to be the boss of your body and what works for you. Don't be taken in by overzealous claims. Don't throw away your good sense of nutrition or your need to establish lifelong healthy habits. Balance your food choices and eat a variety of foods, doing so in moderation. Forget all the crazy options trying to seduce you. Choose to enjoy your food and really love life.

5

It's All About **Me**!
MyPyramid

MyPyramid—Simplified

Me! Me! Me! It's all about me! Well, okay—it's all about you, too! I'm talking about the newest food guide pyramid developed by the United States Department of Agriculture (USDA). The USDA created the first dietary guidelines back in the early 1980s, and those guidelines are updated every five years. This is a good thing because it keeps the guidelines current with the latest nutritional information and probably helps to justify a few jobs. You may recall the media hoopla in 2005 when the old food guide pyramid was laid to rest. This time around the guidelines are called MyPyramid because they get really personal. No, not about your love life but about your personal diet! I'm talking about the fact that one size does not fit all. The new MyPyramid creates a personal eating plan for you with the foods and amounts that are right for you as an individual. Of course, if you have specific health conditions you should consult with your health care provider.

MyPyramid is designed for the general public. You can use this advice to help you make smart choices from every food group, to find your balance between food and physical activity, to get the most nutrition out of your calories, and to stay within your daily calorie needs.

I often recommend the official USDA Web site *www.MyPyramid .gov*—I think it is marvelous! However, I'm in the business. After an intelligent friend told me he had no idea what to do with it, I knew I had to develop a program to help everyday consumers make sense out of it. Let me simplify. I can show you how to implement these guidelines into your life.

Live YOUR *Life*

All adults should strive for at least thirty minutes of moderate physical activity each day. Pick up a pedometer. It's a neat device that can count your individual footsteps. Worn on the hip it clicks with each step. Challenge yourself to increase the number of steps you take each day.

Guidelines Set for Americans: ABCs

The USDA Guidelines can help you understand what you should be eating and how much activity you need to do to stay healthy. People of various cultural backgrounds, age groups, and lifestyles should be able to follow this information. The dietary guidelines describe a healthy diet as one that:

- Emphasizes fruits, vegetables, whole grains, and fat-free or low-fat milk and milk products
- Includes lean meats, poultry, fish, beans, eggs, and nuts
- Is low in saturated fats, trans fats, cholesterol, salt (sodium), and added sugars

Understand that these guidelines are just that—guidelines! These are suggestions to help you stay healthy. They were written to help you achieve and maintain a healthy and active lifestyle. There is also a lot of flexibility so you can make the best food choices for you and the way you live.

At the very least, follow these three basic messages. It's as easy as ABC:

- **A:** Aim for fitness.
- **B:** Build a healthy nutrition base.
- **C:** Choose sensibly.

Aim for Physical Activity!

A woman I know once asked me, "What can I do to up my metabolism rate?" I quickly responded, "get moving!" There is no way around this issue. If you want to drop some pounds and maintain a healthy weight you have got to aim to be physically active.

Finding Your Physical Activities

Physical activity simply means movement of the body while using energy. Walking briskly, climbing the stairs, and even gardening are all considered physical activities. At a minimum you should do activities that add up to at least thirty minutes daily. This is in addition to your usual daily activities. Of course, if you increase the intensity or the amount of time there are additional health benefits and faster weight loss. Do activities that increase your heart rate. Please don't count walking to your refrigerator as being active.

Why Physical Activity?

There are a zillion reasons to be active. It can make you feel better, possibly live longer, and, of course, look great. Following are a few benefits of physical activity.

- Helps to manage your weight
- Improves your fitness level
- Builds muscle strength and improves endurance
- Improves your self esteem
- Helps control blood pressure
- Improves posture and flexibility
- Lowers risk of heart disease, colon cancer, and type 2 diabetes
- Helps build and maintain bones, muscles, and joints
- Reduces feelings of depression

Movement and nutrition work together. Being active helps you to burn more calories. Aging often slows the metabolism down so you need to move more and eat less. Get active!

Build a Healthy Nutrition Base!

Building a healthy nutrition base is the foundation of staying healthy and achieving weight loss. Because no one single food can provide all the nutrients you need, you should consume a number of different foods each day. Here is what you can eat from MyPyramid to get your desired results.

Gravitate to Grains

Foods that are made from wheat, rice, oats, barley, or cereal are considered grains. Think of pasta, bread, and oatmeal, for example. Grain products are low in fat. There are "whole" and "refined" grains. Whole grains contain the entire grain kernel—meaning the bran or germ. Refined grains remove the bran and germ. While milling may lengthen the shelf life of your bread (who wants old bread?), it also removes the dietary fiber, iron, and many B vitamins. The whole truth is whole grains are better!

Cyndi's Secrets™

You can easily increase your fiber intake by keeping peels on your fruits and veggies. A modest baked potato with skin has almost twice the fiber of a "naked" potato the same size.

Vary Your Veggies

There isn't a sensible diet on the planet that disagrees with the importance of eating lots of vegetables. Maybe it's time you took that advice seriously. Whether they are cooked, raw, fresh, frozen, canned, dried, whole, cut-up, or mashed you can't go wrong with vegetables. They are jam packed with nutrients for overall health. They are loaded with fiber, which is great for losing weight. Fiber can help you feel full and eat less. Fiber in your body acts as the roto-rooter of your system and helps to clean you out. MyPyramid recommends five veggie subgroups. These subgroups include vegetables that are dark green, orange, dry beans and peas, starchy vegetables, and all "other" vegetables. Different vegetables provide different nutrients. That's why, to simplify: vary your veggies!

Fruits Are Your Friends

Making friends with fruits is easy. They are delicious. They may be fresh, canned, frozen, or dried. Serve them up whole, cut-up, or puréed. Although 100 percent fruit juice counts as a fruit, make most of your fruit choices whole. My mom used to freeze peach slices from our tree and they were yummy! Just like with vegetables, the nutrients in fruit choices vary. That's why it's wise to make friends with lots of fruits!

Bone-Up on Calcium-Rich Foods

All fluid milk products and many foods made from milk are considered calcium rich. This is important because whether you are two or ninety-two the nutrients in milk build and maintain healthy bones and strong teeth. Choose milk products that retain their calcium content such as all fluid milk, yogurt, or cheese. Avoid foods made from milk that have little or no calcium such as cream cheese, cream, and butter. It is also best to choose fat-free or low-fat milk, yogurt, and cheese. For those who are lactose intolerant, lactose-free products are available.

> **Cyndi's Secrets™**
>
> Fiber acts like a sponge by absorbing water that softens stools and reduces incidence of constipation. It also provides a sensation of fullness by actually slowing the emptying time of the stomach. Fibrous foods are also usually low in fat and calories.

Meat and Beans

Get lean with protein. All foods made from meat, poultry, fish, dry beans or peas, eggs, nuts, and seeds are considered part of this category. If you noticed that "dry beans or peas" are in the vegetable group as well, it's not a typo. Vegetarians are happy that you can kill two birds with one stone—not that we would kill a bird! If you choose meat or poultry, make sure that it is lean or low-fat. It is better to choose fish, nuts, and seeds that contain healthy oils.

Making Peace with Oil

Don't go to war with oil. Some of it is essential. Oils are fats that are liquid at room temperature like cooking vegetable oils. They come from fish and many different plants. Some common oils are canola oil, corn oil, and sunflower oil. Fats that are solid at room temperature such as butter, shortening, or chicken fat come from many animal foods and can also be made from vegetable oils through a process called hydrogenation. Obviously, it's not smart to order a plate of lard. The better fat choices should be from fish, nuts, and vegetable oils. Limit your intake of solid fats like butter, stick margarine, shortening, and lard.

Live YOUR *Life*

Marinate raw veggies in low-calorie Italian dressing. I keep mine covered in the fridge. They make a great healthy snack and help provide lots of vegetable variety.

Use Your Discretionary Calories

What is really cool about MyPyramid is that it allows for the fun food factor. We all have a food weakness. I love chocolate, desserts, and other good stuff. This program gives you a total calorie budget. Your budget can be divided into "essentials" and "extras." If you make smart food choices most of the time there is room in the calorie budget for healthy "little" treats of your choice on occasion. You can call them the "discretionary calories."

Choose Sensibly!

You now know what kind of delicious variety you can have in your diet based on MyPyramid but the trick is you need to choose sensibly. Let me help you sort through some of the food choices that can help you win the battle of the bulge.

Choose a Diet Low in Saturated Fat and Cholesterol

You may be surprised to know that we do need to eat some fat. Fats supply essential fatty acids and help absorb fat-soluble vitamins (vitamins A, D, E, and K) in the body. But problems arise because people tend to eat too much fat. Boy—that's big news! The real big news is you can cut the fat in your diet.

Diets high in fat—particularly saturated fat and cholesterol (both known to increase blood cholesterol levels)—have been linked to heart disease, stroke, obesity, and certain types of cancer. In contrast, consuming fats from unsaturated sources (mainly from vegetable oils) does not raise blood cholesterol levels. You may have also heard about trans fats. Food corporations love these because they extend shelf life, but trans fats are not a good choice and hopefully will be banned soon. Eating too much fat of any type can cause obesity. Your diet should have no more than 35 percent of the total calories coming from fat, and even that is too high for most people. Of this 35 percent, no more than 10 percent should come from saturated fat sources.

Cyndi's Secrets™

Recommendations call for individuals to consume less than 300 milligrams of cholesterol per day. If you eat eggs skip the egg yolk, which has an average of 215 milligrams.

Saturated fats are primarily found in foods from animal sources, like high-fat dairy products (whole milk and cheese), fatty fresh and processed meats, skin and fat on poultry, lard, and also in palm and coconut oils. Cholesterol is also found solely in animal products, primarily in the liver and other organ meats, egg yolks, dairy fats, chicken skin, fatty meats, and in some seafood. Unsaturated fats (which are the better choices) are mainly found in vegetable oils, nuts, olives, avocados, and fatty fish like salmon.

WHAT YOU DON'T KNOW CAN MAKE YOU FAT	Foods high in saturated fats tend to raise blood cholesterol levels. These are found primarily in foods of animal origin. Unsaturated fats do not raise blood cholesterol levels and are found primarily in vegetable sources. Although a wiser choice, these are still 100 percent fat.

In order to follow these recommendations, here's how you can reduce your fat and cholesterol intake:

- Reduce the amount of fat you consume from animal sources, like fat on meats and in milk, butter, cream, and egg yolks.
- Choose lean cuts of meat.
- Remove skin from chicken and poultry before eating.
- Select low-fat dairy products, including milk, yogurt, cheese, and cottage cheese.
- Limit your intake of high-fat convenience snack foods.
- Limit foods like cookies, cakes, pastries, doughnuts, margarine, and cooking oils.
- Become familiar with sources of saturated fat and cholesterol.
- Use liquid cooking spray in place of oil or butter.

- Use whipped butter or "lite" margarine and make sure it has no trans fats.
- Avoid fried foods; opt for baked, broiled, boiled, or grilled foods instead.
- Substitute olive oil, canola oil, or other vegetable oils for solid fats like margarine, butter, or lard.
- Be smart, too, and compare similar products.

Moderate Your Intake of Sugar

Limiting your intake of sugar will likely help you reduce calories, limit your risk of tooth decay, and decrease the incidence of obesity. Sugars can be found in table sugar (sucrose), or in the form of complex sugars like fructose (sugar found in fruit and honey) and lactose (sugar found in milk). Your body cannot tell the difference between the different types of sugars or whether they come from natural or refined sources—all are broken down into glucose during digestion to provide a quick source of energy. Foods high in sugar include white table and brown sugar, honey, molasses, jellies, table syrups, soft drinks, fruit drinks, flavored beverages, candies, and dessert foods. Many of these foods are "discretionary calories." These are foods that offer very few nutrients but a lot of calories. Other foods like potatoes and apples also contain sugar but provide other valuable nutrients as well, so these types of foods

Cyndi's Secrets™

There is no benefit to using honey over sugar. Your body cannot distinguish between table sugar and the complex sugars found in honey, fruit, or milk. It cannot tell whether sugar comes from a natural or refined source.

would not be considered empty discretionary calorie foods. After all, an apple is a better choice as a snack than a candy bar. However, remember that it is okay to "budget" a candy bar on occasion if you choose it as your "extra" calories.

The USDA recommends limiting added sugars in the diet to 6 to 10 percent of total daily calories. (Each teaspoon of sugar equals about 16 calories.) If you eat 1,200 calories per day, that equals no more than 72 to 120 calories from sugar, or 4½ to 7½ teaspoons; if you eat 1,600 calories per day, that means no more than 96 to 160 calories from sugar, or 6 to 10 teaspoons per day; and if you eat 2,200 calories per day, that means no more than 132 to 220 calories from sugar, or 8 to 14 teaspoons.

Sugar is found in obvious food choices, like candies, cookies, cakes, and pastries, but also it can be found in not-so-obvious food choices, like milk, breads, and fruits. But keep in mind that the foods that contain sugar (those empty-calorie foods) and no other nutrition are the ones with which you need to be concerned.

Sources of Sugar

FOOD SOURCE	AMOUNT	TEASPOONS OF SUGAR
Premium cheesecake	1 slice	12
Fruit-flavored beverage	¾ cup	6
Iced cupcake or slice of cake	1	5
Glazed doughnut	1	4
Ice cream	½ cup	4
Chocolate-covered ice cream bar	1	3½
Chocolate-filled sandwich cookies	3	3½
Jelly	1 tbsp.	3
Presweetened cereal	1 cup	3
Fruit leather roll	1	2½

Now, look at some of your favorite foods to see how many teaspoons of sugar they contain. To do so, look at the nutrition facts label, find the grams of sugar, and divide this number by four. In the case of a 12-ounce can of soft drink, we find it has 41 grams of sugar. Divided by four, that equals 10 teaspoons. Wow!

Live YOUR *Life*

Soft drinks are the number one contributor of sugar in the American diet. A 12-ounce can of regular soft drink contributes 10 teaspoons of sugar alone.

Choose and Prepare Foods with Less Salt

Try to limit your salt (or sodium) intake. Too much salt in the diet is linked with high blood pressure. Many foods add salt to the diet, including processed foods, soups, luncheon meats, snack foods, and beverages.

Sodium is important to the body in regulating fluids and blood pressure. Unfortunately, too much sodium in the diet can also cause a person to retain fluids and, as a result, increase the numbers on the scale due to an increase in water weight. It is recommended that you use no more than 2,400 milligrams per day (or 1 teaspoon of salt per day) max.

Check out these tips on reducing your overall salt intake:

- Limit table salt added to foods during preparation.
- Keep your eye open for nutrition labels on processed dinners, convenience foods, crackers, chips, nuts, and seeds, all known to contribute extra sodium.
- Remove the saltshaker from the table. When you shake you have no idea how much is coming out.
- Limit intake of processed foods and luncheon meats.

- Select canned vegetables, soups, and broths without added salt.
- Watch your condiments—ketchup, barbecue sauce, soy sauce, pickles and relish, olives, mustard—all guilty of containing sodium.
- Substitute herbs and spices for salt in flavoring foods.

If You Drink Alcohol, Do So in Moderation

The final dietary guideline offers a message about alcohol consumption. Although not considered a food, alcoholic beverages do contain calories but no other nutrients.

When consumed in large amounts, drinking alcohol can be harmful, even dangerous. A high consumption of alcohol can lead to various health problems including high blood pressure, heart disease, stomach and liver problems, and brain damage. And because of its high calorie content, drinking excessive alcoholic beverages can contribute to obesity. Recommendations continue to suggest limiting consumption to no more than one drink each day for women and two drinks each day for men.

An alcoholic drink refers to any of the following:

- 1 ounce (80 proof) distilled spirits (70 calories)
- 12 ounces regular beer (150 calories)
- 12 ounces light beer (90 calories)
- 4 ounces wine (80 calories)
- 2 ounces sherry (75 calories)

Food Intake Patterns

In the past when you talked about USDA guidelines all one heard over and over again was the reference to "servings." This wasn't a bad approach to portion control but many people just couldn't relate to the term. Nowadays, MyPyramid offers recommendations in cups and ounces and not in servings and serving sizes. You can look at what you eat the whole day rather than how many servings you had during a meal or snack. This is much more user friendly. Of course, the exact amount of food you should consume depends on many factors, including your age, size, gender, health status, and activity level. Young children and teenagers often require additional foods because of their body's needs during the growing years. Athletes may require more servings due to their high energy needs. Sedentary individuals and the elderly often require less because of their less-active lifestyle. And individuals seeking to lose weight may reduce their overall intake.

Go to: *http://www .mypyramid.gov/ professionals/pdf _food_intake.html*

In the corresponding box you will find a link to a graph of the USDA recommended food pyramid— MyPyramid. The food intake graph helps to demonstrate how you can create your personal eating plan coupled with physical activity to achieve healthy balance in your life. However, to really make this work you have to dig deeper. MyPyramid only works if you consume the right amount of each of the food groups for your individual needs. Don't worry, later in this book I show you how to figure out your personal calorie requirements. Once you get that figure flip to the back of the book in Appendix C for some notes on portions.

What's really cool is you can use this table to help you develop healthy food intake patterns that are just right for you. It explains the exact portion sizes that you need without using confusing terms like "servings." Use your calorie requirement calculation and this table to adjust exactly how much of each food group you can eat to reach your personal desired goal.

Promise me that you take a look at this table. It really works! Once you reach your optimum weight goal this table can also help you maintain a healthy weight for life. I love this table. Refer to it often.

Oh, keep in mind that the most effective way to lose weight is to do so with gradual decreases in calorie requirements. This will allow for a slow and steady weight loss. Caloric decreases should be no more than 500–700 calories per day. At this level, individuals can expect a weight loss of about 1 to 2 pounds per week. Get ready to see some smoking results!

Cyndi's Secrets™

You can effectively and safely lose approximately one to two pounds per week by decreasing your calories by no more than 500 to 700 per day. What can you cut back on? Do you really need that soda?

Cater to Yourself

By now you can see that MyPyramid really can cater to you. Decide to make it your own. Try to begin to plan your meals and snacks using the delicious information you have discovered. Choose physical activities that you can do every day.

If you are really ambitious, you can visit *www.MyPyramid .gov.* Click onto the link called MyPyramid Tracker. This is an interactive dietary and physical assessment tool. It helps you evaluate your food choices and physical activity level. It also helps you check out how well you are balancing your energy (calories) consumed with the amount of activity you are doing. In a sense, it helps you keep track of yourself to be sure you are sticking to this program. If you don't take the time to cater to yourself, nobody will.

6 **Taking** the
Pounds Off Plunge

It's My Time

Are you ready to take the pounds off plunge? It's now time to focus on health, good nutrition, and a slow but steady weight loss. Dive in! Ask yourself the following questions:

- Am I ready to make changes to my lifestyle?
- Am I willing to take my time losing weight?
- Do I understand my eating patterns need to be permanent, not temporary?
- Do I understand that the weight will come off slowly?
- Am I willing to increase my activity level?
- Am I willing to plan my meals and snacks?
- Am I motivated to start this time?

If you answered yes to all of these questions, you're ready to begin. Take it slow. Do it right.

Safe Weight Loss—Fun! Fast!

Losing weight safely and effectively requires an approach that includes setting goals (both short-term and long-term goals), changing eating habits, and incorporating physical activity into daily life. Remember: Don't just follow a "diet." Aim to eat healthy!

Re-Set Those Goals

We talked about setting goals at the start of this program. Now that I've given you some rock solid diet information, your next step is to re-set your goals. Make sure they are realistic.

Lose weight for yourself. It's okay to enjoy the appreciation and/or jealousy others might have of you, but it is imperative that you do this for you. Maintain a positive attitude. Remember that short-term goals set your plans for the upcoming week or month—they are attainable. Long-

Live YOUR *Life*

Be realistic. If your goals are too hard you may get frustrated and never meet them.

term goals should not be impossible, but they should challenge and motivate you to keep striving for success. These are goals that you may want to accomplish in six months or a year.

Lose Slowly

Initially your weight-loss goal should be to lose weight slowly. Make small changes. Don't expect drastic results at first. Rome wasn't built in a day. To lose weight slowly, plan to lose no more than one to two pounds each week. You can accomplish this by reducing caloric intake by about 500 calories each day. Here's how. One pound is the equivalent of 3,500 calories. If you want to gain a pound, eat an additional 3,500 calories. If you want to lose a pound, eat a deficit of 3,500 calories. An average person who consumes 2,000 calories per day to maintain his weight would have to increase his caloric intake to 2,500 each day (an additional 500 calories) over a week's time to gain a pound. On the contrary, the opposite is true to lose. This person would have to decrease his caloric intake to 1,500 calories each day (minus 500 calories) over a week's time to lose a pound. Even if you are not good with numbers, like me, you can see that this is very doable. Do it! (Physical activity can also be counted into the equation. The more you move, the more you burn off.)

When you initially use my program to lose weight it's natural to experience some fluid loss. Fluid loss can be as much as one to two pounds but this is only temporary. Continue with the program and you can lose about one to two pounds per week. This is a healthy and adequate weight loss for any person. Just think: If you lost one pound per week for three months you could lose about twelve pounds. In six months, that would make about twenty-five pounds, and in one year, that totals fifty pounds. Think about the last year and reflect on all the so-called diets you have tried. Isn't it now worth the time to do it right and get it off once and for all?

Personalize Your Plan of Attack

Let's face it, none of this information means anything if it doesn't work for you. Take this diet program and make it your own. I like to say I have Cyndified my diet plan. If your name is Bob you can Bobify it, or if you are Barb go ahead and Barbify it. You get the picture. For example, you may think the MyPyramid focuses solely on health and not on weight loss. Wrong!

With the guidelines you can do both if that is what you choose. You might say you can have your cake and eat it too. Well, a small piece.

Your mission is to reduce your food intake while choosing foods from all the groups. Think about balance, variety, and moderation. Select foods that are low in fat and high in fiber. The selections for your personal

plan are endless. Be sure to leave room for a little portion of "discretionary calories."

Taking Little Steps

There are so many ways to cut excess calories from your daily intake that you may be surprised how easy it can be. At first, cutting back 500 calories or so each day may seem extreme, but 50 or 100 calories at a time might be a cut you can easily accomplish. (That's just one cookie or the savings from substituting skim for whole milk.) Here are some other smart alternatives:

- Eat an open-faced sandwich (*1 slice of bread, for savings of 70 calories*)
- Drink black coffee (*1 tsp. sugar and 1 tbsp. cream, for savings of 36 calories*)
- Choose steamed white or brown rice over fried rice (*savings of 100 calories*)
- Substitute light mayonnaise over regular, or, better yet, no mayonnaise (*savings of 65–100 calories*)

- Crunch on ten carrot sticks instead of ten potato chips (*savings of 70 calories*)
- Try plain, low-fat yogurt with added fresh fruit in place of fruited yogurt (*savings of 50 calories)*
- Make a banana smoothie instead of a milkshake (*savings of 50 calories*)
- Snack on a vanilla wafer over a chocolate chip cookie (*savings of 75 calories*)
- Treat yourself with angel food cake, not devil's food cake (*savings of 200 calories*)

Sticking to the Rules

I sometimes enjoy breaking the rules. Not that I am totally rebellious but I love to challenge the norm. It helps me grow as a person. I challenge you to challenge your norm. Try sticking to the guidelines I've proposed in this program and see if you can break out of your old eating patterns. See if you can grow as well—and I'm not talking around the waist. Evolve with your own set of rules using my tips.

Cyndi's Secrets™ for Success

I applaud you for taking the pounds off plunge. Finally you can get this whole weight thing right. I'd like to share some of my personal secrets for weight-loss success. I've used these tips in my own life and with numerous clients. They really work. For more tips, please visit my Web site, *www.starglow.com*, and sign up for my Cyndi's Secrets™ *free* e-tips.

- *Attitude Baby!* If you want results you better think, look, and feel confident!

- *Take teeny steps.* Remember—small, short-term goals can lead to your desired results for life.
- *Plan your meals and snacks.* Write all foods down ahead of time if you need to. Then you will know what to buy and prepare.
- *Eat lots of little healthy meals.* I swear this is the best secret. It makes you want to eat less of the unhealthy choices—sort of a natural appetite suppressant.
- *Plan your portions ahead of time.* This will help control second portions.
- *Take your time eating.* Enjoy the good taste of food. It takes about twenty minutes from the time you begin eating until the time your stomach signals the brain that you're full. By eating slowly, you will often consume less, because you'll begin to feel fuller.
- *Don't skip meals.* This can help you avoid impulse snacking.
- *Sit down when you eat.* Pick a spot, most likely at the kitchen table. I love to curl up on my kitchen counter when I'm in a hurry. It forces me to just "stop" and enjoy the food rather than quickly gobble up more than I need.
- *Fill up on fruits and vegetables.* These high fiber foods make you feel full, so you eat less.
- *If you are full, just stop eating!* You don't have to finish everything in front of you.
- *Keep moving!* Ten minutes here or ten minutes there—it all adds up to weight-loss heaven and health.

7

Consuming Calories **and** Gaining Energy

Defining Calories

A calorie is the amount of energy needed to raise the temperature of a gram of water by 1 degree Centigrade. So what the heck does that mean? Calories (or the energy) in foods are measured by a scientific method called "direct calorimetry." Through this process, foods are actually burned in a chamber surrounded by water to determine how many calories are contained within that particular food. Let me explain what this means to *you*.

Understanding Calorie Counts

Calorie counts are given to foods to show how much food energy they supply. You get this information on nutrition labels found on food products as well as in many books, the Internet, and other resources. It's easy to become obsessed with calorie counts in the foods you eat, without understanding the role they provide in maintaining your life and health.

WHAT YOU
DON'T KNOW
CAN MAKE
YOU FAT
Protein, carbohydrates, and fats (and alcohol) are the only substances that contribute calories or energy to our diets.

Calories are those little buggers that we count, track, eliminate, and discuss all the time. They are used to measure the amount of energy found in food. The more calories a particular food has, the more energy it contains. If calories are energy, you may wonder why we count them to avoid getting fat. Read on.

Balancing Energy Needs

Energy gives us the ability to move, be active, and do work. By understanding your energy needs, you can manage your weight. Your goal should be to know what type of energy goes in and how that energy is used up. The energy in food is measured and counted in calories. When the calories going in your body balance the energy you use going out, body weight is maintained. When the calories going in exceed energy going out, body weight can be gained. And when the calories going in are less than energy going out, body weight can be lost. Basically, the more food energy you eat, the fatter you get unless it is offset by activity. Counting your calorie consumption may seem time consuming at first, but by understanding the definition you can define your waist.

Yummy, Nutrient-Rich Foods

All nutrients are not created equal. There are three main groups of nutrients that contribute calories to our diet: protein, carbohydrates, and fats. Protein and carbohydrates each contribute

4 calories per gram of food. Fat contributes 9 calories per gram of food. Dietary recommendations suggest reducing fat in the diet primarily because fats are so highly concentrated in calories. (Alcohol is not considered a nutrient, but it also contributes calories to the diet at 7 calories per gram.) Foods usually contain a combination of the calorie-contributing nutrients. These nutrients together contribute to that food's total caloric value.

To simplify, let's look at some snacks and see if that helps to illustrate how calories from protein, carbohydrates, and fat work together in one food item. For example, 1 ounce of cheese crackers has 3 grams of protein, 19 grams of carbohydrate, and 7 grams of fat. To determine how many calories the crackers have from protein, multiply the amount of protein (3 grams) times 4 calories/gram, and you see that they have 12 calories from protein. To determine how many calories the crackers get from carbohydrates, take the amount of carbohydrates (19 grams) and multiply it by 4 calories/gram to get 76 calories from carbohydrates. And to determine how many calories the crackers get from fat, multiply the amount of fat (7 grams) times 9 calories/gram to get 63 calories from fat. The total calorie count for the crackers is 151 calories per serving.

On the other hand, a ½ cup of low-fat cottage cheese has 12 grams of protein, 4 grams of carbohydrate, and 2 grams of fat. Multiply the 12 grams of protein times 4 calories/gram, and you see that the cottage cheese has 48 calories from protein. Multiply the 4 grams of carbohydrate times 4 calories/gram, and you see that it has 16 calories from carbohydrate. And multiply the 2 grams of fat times 9 calories/gram, and you get 18 calories from fat, for a total of 82 calories per serving.

Determining Nutrient Percentages

To determine what percentage of each nutrient is in a food product, divide the calories from the nutrient by the total calories. For example, to find the percentage of fat, look at the cheese crackers and cottage cheese again. Determine now what the percentage of fat is in a serving of these foods. To do so, divide the calories from fat by the total calories. So for the cheese crackers, divide 63 calories by 151 calories, and you see that 42 percent of the crackers' calories come from fat. For the cottage cheese, divide 18 calories by 82 calories, and you see that 22 percent of the calories come from fat. You can see from these examples that the cheese crackers are almost half fat while only a fifth of the calories come from fat in the cottage cheese. The cottage cheese contributes a greater amount of protein and less fat than the snack crackers. Hopefully this gives you a smart way to choose better calories for your lifestyle.

Recommendation for Daily Calorie Intake

An overall healthy diet should include a combination of foods that contain protein, carbohydrates, and fats. The Institute of Medicine advises the following Acceptable Macronutrient Distribution Ranges (AMDR) for adults. By combining a variety of foods, you can meet this profile:

- *Protein:* 10 to 35 percent
- *Carbohydrates:* 45 to 65 percent (The majority of these should be complex carbohydrates and no more than 10 percent from simple sugars.)
- *Fat:* 20 to 35 percent (No more than 10 percent should come from saturated fat.)

This program respects your individuality. These guidelines are great because they give you a range to allow for your unique lifestyle and health concerns. Remember, it's all about you! No diet will work unless you make it your own!

Making Friends with Good Carbs

Carbohydrates have been getting a bad rap lately. People are determined to eat fewer of them. The part nobody mentions is that most of the people claiming to lose weight by cutting out the carbs were eating way too many to begin with. Too much of any food is too much, plain and simple.

Carbohydrates primarily include sugars and starches that come from plant sources, along with the natural sugar found in milk. These foods include simple sugars like sucrose (table sugar), fructose (fruit sugar), lactose (milk sugar), and maltose (malt sugar), and complex carbohydrates often referred to as starches. Choose complex carbohydrates because they are loaded with vitamins, minerals and are often lower in fat, calories, and higher in fiber. Additionally, they help the body to maintain normal blood sugar (glucose) levels by promoting a slower, healthier digestion of foods. Starches take longer to digest than sugars. (This is why competitive athletes are encouraged to eat a diet high in complex carbohydrates prior to competition.) You can lose weight and still enjoy an appropriate amount of complex carbs.

Cyndi's Secrets™

If your body doesn't have enough carbohydrates to use for energy, it will use protein (muscles, body tissues, and so on) for the energy it needs. So go get your good carbs!

How Carbohydrates Are Used in the Body

All carbohydrates are broken down during digestion and converted to glucose (blood sugar), where they are then carried to body cells to be used for energy that the body needs. The pancreas then releases insulin to help move the glucose to the cells, where it is burned for energy. If there is more glucose than what the cells need, the remainder is stored in the muscles and liver as glycogen and reserved for later use. If the glycogen stores are full and there is still more glucose, it is then stored as fat. This is why some of the carbohydrate hype is valid for quick weight loss, but read on for the caveat.

Carbohydrates and Weight Reduction. Many people believe that eating carbohydrates is taboo when it comes to weight reducing. This is a total myth. Carbohydrates only become a problem with weight gain when too many and the wrong type are consumed or when preparation methods add excess amounts of fats, like covering pasta (a healthy complex carbohydrate choice) with excess amounts of cream sauce (a not-so-healthy higher-fat choice). Rice with butter, mashed potatoes with gravy, and a bagel with cream cheese are also similar examples of adding fat to a healthy complex carbohydrate food.

Complex carbohydrates are actually the food of choice when seeking to reduce body weight. These foods are highly nutritious, low in fat, and high in fiber. Just don't eat too many of them.

Contribution of Carbohydrates to the Overall Diet. If carbohydrates contribute 55 percent of the total calories in the diet, and a person consumes a 2,000-calorie diet that would equate to 1,100 total calories from carbohydrates. Vegetables, fruits, and grains such as breads, pasta, rice, and cereals, are high in carbohydrates. Legumes (dried beans and peas) are excellent sources as well.

Protein Is Powerful and Important

Nowadays, we hear a lot about protein in the media as if it is a new wonder nutrient. However, it has always been crucial to a balanced diet. It contributes to the development of muscles, bones, cartilage, skin, antibodies, hormones, and enzymes in your body. It is important in the building and maintaining of all bodily structures. It even acts as a source of energy when there are not enough carbohydrates and fats in the diet.

How Protein Is Used in the Body

Protein is built by a combination of chemical structures called "amino acids." There are about twenty amino acids that the body needs, and these are often referred to as the building blocks of body. Of the twenty amino acids, nine are essential to the diet, meaning they must be supplied by the foods we eat. The remaining amino acids can be made in the body. When a food is consumed that includes all nine of the essential amino acids, it is referred to as a complete protein source. Meat, poultry, fish, eggs, and dairy products like milk and cheese all are complete protein sources. Incomplete sources of protein are those that do not contain the amount of essential amino acids needed by the body. These sources are primarily fruits and vegetables. But some plant sources offer some of the essential amino acids while others offer the remaining ones.

Cyndi's Secrets™

Rice and beans can be eaten at different times of the day and still make up a complete protein.

If you are a vegetarian, this is particularly important. You want to be sure you get your complete proteins. This can be accomplished by combining various sources of plant proteins with each other, therefore adding up to a complete protein. For example, if rice is consumed with beans, this combination becomes a complete protein source. For more menu selections, pick up *The Everything® Vegetarian Cookbook*.

Protein Requirements

The amount of protein needed by a person is based on age, sex, and body size. The recommended dietary allowance for protein in adult males over twenty years of age ranges from 58 to 63 grams per day. For adult females over twenty, the allowance ranges from 46 to 50 grams per day. Most people do not have trouble meeting protein requirements. In fact, many often consume up to twice as much.

Protein and Weight Reduction

Many people are into high-protein weight-reduction diets. They may have found that these high-protein diets can lead to weight loss. But excess protein in the diet is not a wise choice. Too much protein (and in many cases the excess fat that results) can lead to risk of health problems along with a condition called "ketosis." By not having enough energy from carbs, the body starts using protein for energy. This makes your liver and kidneys work extra hard. You may not notice it right away, but this condition can be harmful in the long run. This is one reason that consuming excess protein through high-protein diets is not a healthy way to lose weight. Besides, many people on a high-protein diet are already eating more protein than their diet recommends.

Contribution of Protein to the Overall Diet

Protein should account for about 10 to 35 percent of total daily calories. For a person consuming a 2,000-calorie diet, with 15 percent from protein, this would equate to about 300 total calories. A variety of lean meats, poultry, fish, eggs, low-fat dairy products, and dried beans and peas should contribute to this intake.

You Can Eat Fat

Fat often conjures up negative feelings. Certainly too much fat is linked to health problems like heart disease, stroke, obesity, and some types of cancers. But, in fact, fats are an essential part of all cells in the body. Fat helps maintain the health of the skin and hair, transports fat-soluble vitamins (vitamins A, D, E, and K) throughout the body, cushions the body organs to keep them safe from injury, and serves as a protective insulator to the body on cold days.

In addition, fats contribute to the taste, smell, and texture of foods as well as providing a satiety factor of fullness after eating foods that contain it. The reason fats take so long to digest is because they are so calorie dense, containing 2.5 times the number of calories that are found in carbohydrates and protein. But in order to meet your body's need for fat, you should aim to eat foods with the right type and amount of fat.

The Various Types of Fat

Understanding fats can be confusing. We often hear the terms "good" and "bad" fats. I use them too. In fact, the fat in my diet is primarily made up of "good" fats but I have the "bad" fats on occasion as part of my "discretionary calories."

Don't you just love those? Following is a list of the various types of fat.

Monounsaturated and Polyunsaturated Fats: These are called the good fats. Think of salmon, tuna, olives, avocados, canola oil, walnuts, and peanut oil.

Saturated Fats and Trans Fats: These are the bad guys. Foods with this type of fat include butter, margarine, ice cream, beef, processed foods, and mayonnaise.

The differences between these types of fats are a result of their chemical makeup. The more hydrogen the chemical makeup contains, the more saturated the fat becomes. It is also possible to distinguish some fats by their appearance. Saturated fats are those that are typically solid at room temperature, like lard, butterfat, and beef fat (the fat marbled throughout meat).

WHAT YOU DON'T KNOW CAN MAKE YOU FAT	Don't be fooled by coconut oil, palm oil, and palm kernel oil. These fats are an exception. They may be liquid vegetable oils, but they are actually saturated fats that can increase health risks of heart disease and cancer.

The bad trans fats are making headlines regularly. They are made up of polyunsaturated oils that are saturated with hydrogen atoms. Food companies love these because they help extend the shelf life of a food product. They have often been labeled as hydrogenated or partially hydrogenated, which is very misleading. New laws are forcing corporations to label food products as having trans fats and to not use them at all. I wish trans fats would disappear from the planet. Try not to use these at all, even as your "discretionary calories."

Health risks are primarily associated with diets high in saturated or trans fats and are known to increase overall risk of heart disease and some types of cancer. Unsaturated and polyunsaturated fats are usually from plant sources and are liquid or soft at room temperature. These fats can actually help decrease health-related problems and reduce risk factors of heart disease and various types of cancers.

Cholesterol

Cholesterol is not a fat but is often categorized with fats. It's a white, waxy substance found in animal products. It builds tissues and cell walls, and it is required for the manufacturing of hormones and bile. Cholesterol, a component of many foods like butter, egg yolk, meat fat, poultry skin, organ meats, and shellfish, is also made in the body. Because of health concerns with excessive consumption, cholesterol should be limited to 300 milligrams or less per day.

Cyndi's Secrets™

Cholesterol is found only in animal tissues. Therefore, foods containing it must come from an animal source. Foods like peanut butter cannot contain cholesterol.

Fat and Weight Control

For most Americans, cutting back to 20 to 35 percent or less of total calories from fat is a suggested goal, with 10 percent or less of this total coming from saturated fat. But it is not necessary to track the percentage of every kind of fat you eat. Instead, a simpler method would be to watch those fat grams. A diet that combines a variety of foods, both higher and lower in fat, in moderate portions helps to provide the variety and balance you need.

Meeting Your Caloric Needs

Although you don't have to think about calories 24/7, it is really helpful to understand approximately how many calories it takes for your body to function. This will, in turn, help you to estimate how much you need to reduce your intake of foods in order to lose weight. Once you establish your caloric needs, refer to that fabulous food intake table on the MyPyramid Web site. This can help you tremendously in establishing your personal plan of action. What are you waiting for? Get calculating—it's fun! Knowing what you are up against is the first step and an important part of the battle.

Resting Metabolic Needs

To determine the number of calories you need to lose weight, you first need to estimate the number of calories you need to maintain your body weight—your body weight at its current level. First you must establish how many calories it takes to maintain your normal body functions at rest. This is referred to as your basal metabolic rate (BMR). Once you determine this number, then you will be able to add additional calories to compensate for daily activities and needs for basic body functions. I'll show you how. Start with this equation:

To determine your BMR, multiply your current weight by ten (for women) or eleven (for men).

A 150-pound woman has a BMR of 1,500. This is the approximate amount of energy (calories) that this individual needs at rest. (Although BMR is primarily calculated from kilogram weight, this formula will still provide you with an accurate estimate of your needs without converting weight to kilograms.)

Activity Needs

Because your body does more than just rest, and because you need energy (calories) to meet physical needs, you must further determine your activity needs.

To determine your activity needs do the following.

- If you are mostly sedentary during the day (sitting, standing, reading, writing, and not doing much physical activity), multiply your BMR by 0.20.
- If you are lightly active during the day (doing housework, playing with children, walking two miles or less during the course of the day), multiply your BMR by 0.30.
- If you are somewhat active during the day (doing heavy housework or gardening, playing tennis, working out at a club, dancing), multiply your BMR by 0.40.
- If you are very active during the day (working in construction, doing heavy labor, playing team sports regularly), multiply your BMR by 0.50.

So our lightly active, 150-pound woman, with a BMR of 1,500, would multiply 1,500 by 0.30. Her adjustment for activity needs would be 450. That means she needs 1,500 calories just to get by without any physical activity, but she needs another

450 calories on top of that to accommodate her activity. Her total BMR would be 1,500 plus 450, or 1,950 calories.

Basic Digestive/Absorption Needs

About 10 percent of your daily calories are needed to meet basic digestive/absorption functions. Take your total BMR (with activity factored in) times 0.10. So the woman from the last section, with a total BMR of 1,950, would multiply 1,950 by 0.10, to get 195. Add that to 1,950, and you see she needs 2,145 calories to maintain her current weight.

This formula is just a guideline for people to determine their approximate BMR. There are many factors that contribute to it as well. Besides gender differences, BMR is also affected by heredity and body composition.

Cyndi's Secrets™

Metabolism is defined as all the work your body does that uses calories—the work needed to stay alive, think, breathe, and move. And your BMR is a result of your daily basal metabolic needs (about 60 to 70 percent), your daily activity needs (about 20 to 30 percent), and your daily digestion/absorption needs (about 10 percent).

It's Not Always Your Fault

Fast or slow metabolisms can be inherited. (Wouldn't we all love to have a fast metabolism?) This is why some people stay thin throughout their life while eating whatever they desire, while others feel like the pounds just pile on. Your body composition is also a factor in determining your BMR. Some people's bodies have more muscle, others more bone, while yet others have more fat. A person who is muscular and lean will have a higher metabolism than someone built with a larger amount of fat. Muscle burns more energy (calories) than fat does. So the more muscle you have, the more calories you will burn. This is why it is so important to build those muscles throughout life.

Differences Between Men and Women

Women are prone to burning fewer calories than men. This is a fact. It's because a woman's body contains a higher percentage of fat than a man's body. It may not seem fair, but, again, it is what it is. Men usually have 10 to 20 percent more muscle than women do, and therefore burn calories at a higher rate. Women's bodies have increased fat stores to help them compensate for times of special need during their lives, such as during pregnancy and lactation.

Losing One Pound at a Time

Let me show you how many calories are necessary to begin to lose weight in a healthy manner. As stated in the last chapter, 3,500 calories equal one pound. To lose one pound, you need to decrease your caloric intake by 3,500 calories. You can see from the above example that it is not possible to put your body in a deficit of 3,500 calories within the course of a day or two. Decreasing your calories sufficiently by 500 calories per day you can lose one pound per week (500 calories multiplied by seven days equals 3,500 calories). The idea is to create a negative energy balance—consume fewer calories than you use up without sacrificing your other nutrient needs. This will allow for a weight loss of about one pound per week. If you want to lose fast this may seem too low for you. But this approach will help you to lose body fat (not muscle or water weight), incorporate a healthier food intake, and achieve permanent results. As you begin to lose weight, you can also increase your activity levels to burn even more calories. This will help burn more calories and guess what? You lose the weight faster.

Starting Over at Any Age

I don't want to hear the age-old excuse—*age*—when it comes to your weight loss. Sure, you may have to adjust to normal changes in the body but you can do it. One obstacle when it comes to getting older is the decline of metabolic rate. There is an energy reduction of 3 to 5 percent that occurs each decade (after twenty-five to thirty years of age). This happens because of changes such as body composition and hormones. Bodies become less active. Muscle tissue declines. Body fat increases. With less overall muscle mass, fewer calories are burned for normal energy needs.

> **Cyndi's Secrets™**
>
> Unless you exercise regularly, your metabolism can decrease as much as 3 to 5 percent each decade during your adult life. So, no matter what your age, get a move on!

This does not have to be depressing. There are countless studies and examples of people living today who are in better shape now than when they were younger. Exercise and physical activity can help increase your muscle tissue to accelerate your metabolism and calorie needs. By working out your major muscle groups twice each week you can help replace a decade's loss of muscle mass in several months. Wow! So lift those weights and build your strength to help reduce the aging process. It can make you feel younger and stronger and can improve your sex life, too.

Reasons for Weight Gain

People over twenty-five and up to sixty-five years of age often experience weight gain due in part to aging. However, even young people beginning a professional career just after high school or college often become more sedentary. Weight gain can creep up here and there until a few pounds turn into an overweight or obese condition.

As lifestyles become more affluent, so do higher standards of living, which can mean doing fewer chores. If you hire people to clean your house, cut your grass, or wash your cars, you may save yourself from doing the work but you burn fewer calories. People also eat out more often, enjoy social eating events, and spend more money on food overall. Each one of these can contribute to weight gain over the years.

Do People Have a Predetermined Weight?

You may notice that some people can maintain their weight without a great deal of effort while others fight to lose beyond a certain point. Many nutrition scientists believe in a theory often referred to as the set point theory.

A set point is a weight range that your body aims to maintain. It is based on your genetic and chemical makeup. Your body works hard to stay within a minimal range surrounding this set point. The body's metabolism decreases when weight drops lower than its set point so weight loss is slow; on the contrary, it increases when weight rises above the set point. The body works hard to keep this balance. Set points are often noticed when comparing two people of the size height and same frame size. Even if these two people ate the same foods, they would not necessarily gain weight the same way or lose weight the same way. The weight they carry is dependent on their genetic makeup and ultimately on their set point. The set point theory can explain many mysteries surrounding weight reduction and dieting.

Energy-Ease

The energy needs of individuals are different. Yours are unique, too, based on various factors. Determining your particular needs can help you estimate a guideline within which to work. Body size, metabolism, age, gender, activity levels, and genetics all are factors in establishing one's exact energy needs. Rather than focusing on a specific number, instead try to understand where your energy is coming from and how you can aim to properly meet individual food energy requirements. This can be much more effective in losing and maintaining your overall weight.

8

Move It **or**
Lose It!

Fun Fit Facts

What do you know about exercise and physical fitness? Let's test you. Answer the following true-or-false questions:

1. In order to reap the benefits of exercise you need to push yourself to your limits.
2. If you sweat more, you will lose more weight.
3. Exercising will make you eat more overall.
4. The best option for losing weight would include a combination of aerobic conditioning and strength training.
5. It doesn't pay to begin an exercise program as a senior citizen if you have never exercised before in your life.
6. Spot reducing is the best way to tackle a problem with fat on a particular part of the body.
7. Cellulite has nothing to do with your body fat.

Here are the answers:

1. **False.** Excessive exercise can actually do more harm than good. Pushing yourself too hard increases risk of injuries to the bones, joints, and muscles and can also make you dislike exercising altogether. If you are overdoing your workouts, you would benefit more from slowing it down, enjoying what you are doing, and making exercise a part of your everyday routine. But fess up—do you even come close to being an excessive exerciser?

2. **False.** Water weight can be lost through excess perspiration but this is only temporary. Once fluids are reintroduced to the body, this water weight will return. When exercising, replace fluids on a regular basis.

3. **False.** It is true that some people experience variations in their appetite, but, on the whole, regular exercise should not increase or decrease your appetite.

4. **True.** You can lose weight more quickly and effectively when you do both aerobics and strength training regularly. Doing aerobic activities burns more calories than doing strength training, which builds more muscle. However, having stronger muscles helps your body work more efficiently to burn more calories when you do your aerobics.

5. **False.** Don't even think of using the age excuse! People of all ages can benefit from an exercise program. Even a simple regular walking program can be of great benefit. If you are a senior, get involved in a regular fitness routine. By doing so, you can gain muscle mass and improve strength, flexibility, and endurance. Many seniors who suffer from elevated blood sugar levels as a result of non-insulin-dependent dia-

betes and high blood pressure have seen those levels come down after starting a workout program. If Mick Jagger can rock the super bowl as a senior, then you can take the dog for a walk and get some satisfaction in the pounds you lose.

6. **False.** You cannot spot reduce. Fat doesn't just melt off one part of your body. However, you can tone the muscles underneath your fat. Cardiovascular fitness helps to burn the fat, while doing strength exercises, such as sit-ups for the abs or leg presses for your thighs, can help you define and firm up your shape. The best way to lose that flabby stomach or trim those thighs is to do both aerobics and strength training.

7. **False.** Cellulite and body fat are one and the same. Cellulite is just fat with a dimply appearance, which comes from the way it is deposited in the body. Again, weight loss through a plan of reduced calories and fat combined with an increase in exercise will help combat or at least reduce the appearance of cellulite.

Live YOUR *Life*

Don't be insecure about cellulite. I've known and worked with centerfold models who have it. It is often touched up for these ladies. If only we all could have that luxury!

Get Off the Couch!

Do you spend your life sitting around? Boring! Boring! Get out there and shake some booty. Do some form of exercise or physical activity that you truly enjoy. And if you think you just won't like anything, try something new. Just move! For example, I am a kick boxer, but once when I broke my toe it was tough. I started swimming, which was new for me, and realized that although the chlorine was a little rough on my blonde hair, I had fun, got a great workout, and discovered a really good hair conditioner. Exercise or physical fitness and activities of all types contribute to an active lifestyle. The more you move, the healthier you are.

Isn't It Worth the Effort?

There are tons of activities you can do to help change your sedentary lifestyle into an active one. Join an aerobics or step class; go biking, swimming, jogging, skiing, skating, or even dancing. If you are afraid of being a klutz there is always spinning. This is a fun class on a bike where you can adjust the resistance to simulate riding up and down hills without the worry of tripping on your feet. Try a team sport like tennis, softball, football, or basketball. They say if your dog is fat you're not getting enough exercise. How about giving fat Fido a walk around the block? You both can benefit. Any and all activities add up. Determine what you like to do and build a daily program.

Weight Loss and Maintenance

Body weight is regulated by the number of calories consumed. By doing physical activity, you can lose those extra calories that would otherwise be stored as fat in your body. When more calories are consumed than are used for energy, weight gain occurs. When more calories are burned for energy than are consumed, weight loss occurs. Balancing consumed calories with burned ones results in weight maintenance. I can't say enough about it! Burning up extra calories by being active leads to weight loss. Strenuous activities like running, dancing, and biking help burn more calories than more moderate activities like walking and gardening, but it all adds up. See how your favorite activity ranks in the chart below. To calculate the approximate number of calories burned from each activity, multiply the number listed by your weight and then by the number of minutes spent doing each activity.

ACTIVITY	APPROXIMATE CALORIES/MINUTE
Dancing, aerobic	0.077
Dancing, ballroom	0.023
Fishing	0.029
Gardening	0.036
Mopping floors	0.028
Mowing grass	0.051
Playing piano	0.018
Playing drums	0.035
Raking leaves	0.025
Running, 8 minute/mile	0.100
Running, 6 minute/mile	0.127
Scrubbing floors	0.049
Shoveling snow	0.060
Sitting/reading	0.010
Swimming, fast	0.073
Swimming, slow	0.059
Yard volleyball	0.044
Walking leisurely	0.036
Walking up hills	0.055
Washing car	0.026

Let's say a 150-pound person wants to know how many calories were burned in a sixty-minute walk. Multiply 150 (for weight) by 0.036 (for activity) by 60 (for minutes spent exercising). The result tells us that 324 calories were burned.

There are many benefits to exercise, including:

Increase in Energy Levels. Many people are afraid that exercise is going to make them too tired. However, exercise can increase your energy.

Psychological Improvements. It is a fact that people who exercise regularly feel better about themselves, have greater self-confidence and energy, handle stress better, and are less likely to be depressed than those who don't work out.

Increased Social Opportunities. Joining an exercise class, fitness club, golf foursome, tennis league, or sports team offers many opportunities to meet people, enjoy the company of others, and keep active. Be a team player and see how much you can gain. I have to admit I have met some cute guys with a zest for life at the gym. Although there were some dumbbells, too, and I don't mean weights.

> ### Cyndi's Secrets™
>
> Drink several ounces of water every twenty minutes during exercise. If the weather conditions are warm, water should be consumed every ten to fifteen minutes.

Enjoying Your Activities

There are many types of activities available to you. Obviously whatever you choose, you should enjoy. But some exercises offer greater benefits than others do.

Aerobic Conditioning

If you want to cut through the fat fast there is nothing like a good aerobic workout. An aerobic or cardiovascular activity uses oxygen to increase the blood circulation. This makes your heart pump harder and become more efficient. In addition to trimming off the fat, there are tremendous benefits from safely getting your heart rate up. You can expect to feel better and improve your overall general health. It can lower blood pressure, strengthen the lungs, lower cholesterol, and help prevent heart disease and other medical illnesses. The energy aerobics can give you is dynamic.

Live YOUR *Life*

Now is a great time to be active! Join a ballroom dance class or bowling league. Try my new Cyndi's Secrets™ DVD workout series (starglow.com) or my CD, *Drive to Fitness*, for moves you can do in your car, home, or office. It's fun!

I have often said that if most people would give it a try they would never want to quit. The high from a good aerobic workout can help you manage stress better. For maximum benefits, do some form of aerobics three times a week for a minimum of twenty to thirty minutes, moving your large muscles at an even pace. Some aerobic activities include jogging, fast walking, biking, dancing, skating, and skiing. It is important

WHAT YOU DON'T KNOW CAN MAKE YOU FAT

Aerobic means "with oxygen" and denotes activities where oxygen demand can be met continuously during performance, such as walking or jogging. Anaerobic means "without oxygen" and denotes activities where the muscles are using oxygen faster than the heart and lungs can deliver it. These activities include quick stop-and-go movements, like in baseball, and tennis. You'll need plenty of both to be in shape.

to monitor your heart rate to keep your workout both safe and effective.

Later in the chapter I'll show you how to determine your target heart rate and how this knowledge enhances your workout.

Everyday Moderate Activities

Everyday moderate activities that are low in intensity may not be considered aerobic but are still very beneficial. Consider doing activities such as gardening, cleaning house, raking leaves, mowing the grass, playing with children, and leisurely walking to help you keep moving. Although these activities may not seem that you are doing much, they are just as important as aerobic activities for overall health and weight maintenance. Accumulation of these types of activities adds up to more calories burned overall. Remember that you need to accumulate at least thirty minutes of activity a day for MyPyramid to work.

Strengthening Exercises

Exercises that include weight bearing or resistance training should also be a part of your exercise routine. Resistance training helps strengthen muscles and bones; improves overall conditioning, endurance, and balance; and assists in preventing injuries. Strength-training exercises should be incorporated into regular exercise programs at least twice per week. You want to be sure to

| WHAT YOU DON'T KNOW CAN MAKE YOU FAT | Muscle weighs more than fat, so building up muscle can initially add a few pounds rather than taking them off, but in time this will reverse. So go for the burn! Muscle sure is better than fat, isn't it? |

work on all your major muscle groups in the upper body, lower body, and core. The core includes the abs and your lower back.

Even walking is considered a form of resistance training. If you don't have weights you can use cans, water bottles, or inexpensive stretchy tubing.

Flexibility Exercises

Exercises that improve flexibility such as stretching, yoga, and Pilates are those that help to move your joints in all areas of motion. You really need to stretch if you want to prevent injuries. If you have any aches and pains in your joints, stretching can help you to move your body more freely. Stretch the muscles in your shoulders, knees, elbows, hips, and ankles. I even stretch my toes. Stretching helps elongate the muscles and connective tissues. Hold each stretch for at least twenty to thirty seconds. Do not bounce but *hold* the stretch. Stretch whenever you can. I do in front of the TV, in my car, right now as I'm writing, and at the gym. Experts have conflicting opinions as to whether you should stretch before or after strength training. I favor a five-minute cardio warm-up, followed by my workout, and ending with a stretch.

Rest, Relax, Reduce

For optimum workout results you have to rest. I don't mean take a nap in the middle of your home workout. Wouldn't that be a nice treat? Follow these suggestions:

- Make sure you get your sleep so that the body functions at its best.
- Never work the same muscle group two days in a row with weights. For example, if you worked the chest and back on

Wednesday you would rest those muscles on Thursday. On Thursday you could choose to work other muscle groups such as the lower body. It is on the day of recovery that the strengthening and firming really occurs.

• Be sure to rest in between sets of repetitions. If you do eight arm curls, stop and rest for thirty seconds before you do the next set of eight.

Getting Started—Less Is More

Every exercise program should begin with a plan. Whether you decide to work out in a gym, in your home, or start a walking program, the best success lies with a program that is incorporated into daily schedules. A common pitfall is to do too much, which can lead to muscle pain and burnout. When getting started, less is more. You need to be committed, motivated, and also enjoy what you are doing in order to gain benefits over the long haul.

Evaluate Your Health

If you have not had a recent physical examination or are over the age of sixty, you should see your doctor before you begin a regular fitness program. It is always a wise idea. Your doctor can determine if you have any health-related problems that need to be observed, such as heart problems, chest pains, high blood pressure, diabetes, or arthritis.

Begin Slowly

When starting an exercise program, always go at your own safe pace. I give my clients a little less to do at first. It helps to avoid injury and leaves them wanting more. The idea is to gradually challenge you. The results are more effective and your enthusiasm to move can last a lifetime.

Get Your Gear

I regularly prowl the floors of fitness conventions searching for the latest and the best in fitness gear. At the top of my list are workout shoes. They aren't just sneakers anymore. You can choose a pair for your specific activity or get cross-trainers for all your activities. Make sure they fit. Workout clothes need to be functional and comfortable. Okay, and cute, too, if you choose. If you are walking or jogging outdoors, wear layers so you can adapt to weather changes. Most experts recommend loose clothes but I say get clothes that are comfortable and "fit." It's too easy to think like a fat person and eat too much in super baggy clothes. Wear workout gear that makes you look and feel your best.

Sneakers may be the most important things. When you're buying sneakers, keep in mind the following suggestions:

- Try on several different brands and sizes before making a selection.
- Shop later in the day when feet are most likely swollen.
- Try shoes on with athletic socks. Tie snugly.
- Make sure both shoes fit. Sometimes one foot may be slightly larger.
- Don't just walk around in the store. Run, skip, jump, and mimic your favorite physical activity. What good is an expensive shoe on the store floor if it cramps your toes when you play basketball?

Choose Activities You Enjoy

An exercise routine is good only if it's followed regularly. You should enjoy what you do. Try a dance class or join a walking group. Choose whatever you like, whatever keeps you going. Try watching television while walking on a treadmill or while pedaling on a stationary bike. Or read a juicy novel. Also, what about that video game trend? I love the dancing games—it's a great workout for the entire family, right in your living room.

Make a Schedule

Just as you should plan your meals and snacks, it is important to plan your activities. Put fitness dates on the calendar just like you would do for a meeting or appointment.

Alternate Your Routine

Select a variety of activities you enjoy to avoid boredom and to ensure that you stimulate different muscle fibers. If you walk or bike regularly, choose different routes. If you go to a fitness club, try different group classes or equipment on different days of the week. At home, switch from the treadmill to jumping rope.

Live YOUR *Life*

Boredom is the number one reason that many people stop exercising. If your exercise routine is too boring, find something else.

Find a Friend

People often succeed with workout buddies. It keeps the workout fun. Friends (and family members) who join efforts offer encouragement to keep you motivated. And what a great way to visit with others! Just make sure they truly are good buddies and not friends who secretly want you to be heavier than they are out of insecurity. Unfortunately, this seems to happen all the time.

Challenge Yourself

Throughout this whole program I have stressed the importance of setting goals for your diet. It's just as important to set workout goals. Establishing both short- and long-term goals can help to challenge and inspire you.

Enter the Healthy Heart Rate Zone

If you want to lose weight quickly and safely, you need to enter the healthy heart rate zone during your cardio workout. This is the range where your heart and lungs get the best and safest workout. Your training heart rate range should be between 60 and 85 percent of your maximum heart rate. Maximum heart rate is the highest heart rate you can achieve during vigorous exercise.

First, calculate your maximum heart rate by subtracting your age from 220. For example, if you are forty years old, your maximum heart rate is 180 (220 minus 40).

You also need to check your pulse during exercise. This allows you to count the number of times your heart beats and to monitor the intensity of the workout. Place your index and middle fingers—don't use your thumb, as it has its own pulse—either on your wrist or neck. While watching the second hand on a clock, count the number of beats for ten

Cyndi's Secrets™

Just when you think you've had enough water to drink, have some more. A person's thirst mechanism is not a good indicator of the body's need for fluids, and drinking the extra fluid allows for sufficient intake.

seconds. Multiply this number by six to determine the number of beats per minute.

The following chart shows you where your target heart rate zone should be for your age. If you are a beginner, your workout should be at the lower end of the range, around 55 to 60 percent or 108 to 135 beats per minute. If you are advanced you can workout at a higher intensity up to 85 percent of maximum heart rate.

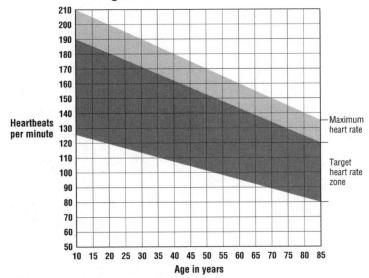

Target Heart Rate for Exercises

You should aim to exercise within a safe target heart rate zone. This zone is the range in which your heart is obtaining an effective workout. Varying with ages and fitness abilities, this zone is a range between a person's resting heart rate and their maximum heart rate. When you begin a fitness program, aim for the lower end of your zone; then seek to increase it as your ability increases.

Cyndi's Top Tips to Motivate

Need help in getting motivated to move? Follow my top tips:

- *Make fitness a priority.* If you have time to eat, then you can find time to squeeze in a workout. Even ten-minute sessions are advantageous.
- *Respect your body type.* Whether you are apple- or pear-shaped, there are limits to what you can achieve. Be realistic in the drive to be fit.
- *Love yourself naked.* Look in the mirror and like what you see before you begin. Love yourself enough to embrace exercise.
- *Go for goals.* Short- and long-term goals are needed for fitness. Make these at the same time you set your diet goals. Write them in your diary.
- *Establish a mental and physical plan.* Use your mind over your body as you focus on your workout challenges in the present. I say enjoy the journey!
- *Use the power of positive visualization.* Take a few minutes each day and visualize what you can look and feel like when you reach your goals. Know this is a lifetime commitment.
- *Improve your body age.* You can't change your chronological age, but you can slow down the aging process.
- *Be prepared for setbacks.* They happen to everyone. Pick yourself up by your bootstraps and go forward!

9

Staying On **Track—** Eating Well

Eating Out Challenges

The American lifestyle is fast and it's changing constantly. We have crazier schedules than ever before. Family meals at home are nearly extinct. No longer do dads come home by 6:00 P.M. to their family and a hot meal waiting at the table. No longer do moms stay home slaving over the stove. For that matter, the kids aren't home anyway because of their various after-school activities. Breakfast today is often quick, easy, and grabbed on the way out the door. Lunches are typically packed or picked up at work, school, or at the diner. And dinner? Well, that's up for grabs in most families, depending on the day of the week. Weekends do offer a little extra time for many families to be together at mealtime.

You Can Eat Out and Lose Weight

The trend to eat out is not going to stop. Although we should all try to eat at home more often, I'd be a hypocrite if I told you to stop eating out altogether. Admittedly, reviewing a restaurant menu comes with challenges when trying to lose weight. However, what I love about my program is that you can eat out and lose weight.

WHAT YOU DON'T KNOW CAN MAKE YOU FAT	The frequency of eating out has risen by more than 66 percent in the last two decades. Current estimates are that Americans eat more than a quarter of total meals out of the house.

Monitor the Times You Eat Out

It is difficult to keep track of extra calories and large portions when you eat out. Let's face it—you don't have total control over what goes into restaurant food. Try to monitor the times you eat out. This is particularly important if you are trying to lose weight. Rather than inadvertently running into a restaurant at the last minute with starvation pangs, plan for those times each week when you want to eat out. On the flip side, plan meals that you can prepare for yourself. For example, during the week you can plan to pack yourself one or two breakfasts or lunches instead of eating out every day. This can help you manage your food intake better.

Live YOUR *Life*

For most people, eating out occasionally will not cause a problem with a healthy lifestyle. It all depends on what is ordered and what is eaten.

Select Restaurants That Offer Choices

There are so many restaurants available to you. Choose with care. If someone else selects the restaurant, order extra carefully.

In any case, try to frequent restaurants that offer a wide variety of foods and preparation methods. And, by all means, do not be afraid to speak up! Ask servers how the food is cooked. If it is not to your liking, talk to the chef about making a special request. I get so specific when I order that I often get lovingly teased.

Remember, you are a paying customer. Most chefs are happy to please you. If not, don't frequent those restaurants. It's smart to care about what types of foods go into your body and how they are prepared.

Make Healthy Menu Selections

Look for menu items that are low in fat. Stay away from fried, batter-dipped, and creamy foods. You can often substitute fresh fruits and vegetables for French fries, hash browns, or potato chips. I order my veggies steamed with no butter. They are less soppy that way and taste better. Order your salad with the dressing on the side. If you have turkey or roast beef, the gravy should also be on the side. This way you can control how much is poured on top. Avoid extra butter or margarine. It adds up quickly.

Baked potatoes are very nutritious. However, order them plain instead of stuffed with butter and sour cream.

Cyndi's Secrets™

If the salad dressing you ordered on the side comes in a gravy bowl, don't eat the whole serving. One level tablespoon or less is plenty.

Watch the bread basket, too. Does it make sense to eat a loaf of sourdough bread slathered with butter before you gobble up your sandwich? This can double or triple the amount of bread you consume.

Watch Your Portions

A big part of the success of this program is portions. I should say "a small part," because it is small portions that can help you lose and maintain your weight. Some meals are actually four to six times the recommended serving size. Many people like to be served big portions in restaurants because they feel they get what they pay for. However, when your waist size gets bigger it's an even bigger price to pay. When you are eating out and that huge, delicious fish or chicken dish is sitting in front of you, the temptation is staring you in the face. Stop for a second and tell yourself that you do not have to finish it. Take some home for another meal. Make a split down the middle of your meal before you even start eating. If it helps, you can even put half away in a doggie bag before you start to eat. Out of sight, out of mind. You can even share your meal with someone else. This is really romantic on a date. Many guys I have dated have thanked me for the weight they lost just because I encouraged sharing.

| WHAT YOU DON'T KNOW CAN MAKE YOU FAT | Watch out for the latest trap in advertising. It's called "The Fourth Meal." You don't need a complete extra entrée at the end of the night that's processed and loaded with fat. Stay away from fast food at midnight, and no, that chocolate cake in the fridge is not calling your name! |

Try Desserts Occasionally

I love desserts! That is one of my weaknesses and may be yours too. If so, do what I do and opt for a healthier choice. Try fresh fruit, sherbet, or angel food cake topped with fresh strawberries. These satisfy the sweet tooth and taste great too!

Of course a "little" portion of dessert is okay as long as it's part of your "discretionary calories."

The Nation of Fast Food

Fast-food restaurants are everywhere. Whether you are single or married, and certainly if you have kids, fast food is convenient and usually inexpensive. I don't recommend you frequent these restaurants often. They are havens for overly processed food and double doses of excess fat. However, to be realistic, I know a drive-through is probably in your future. Just try to limit the number of times you eat at them. Be sure to balance fast-food meals with other foods lower in fat and calories throughout the day.

To keep your diet in line, stay away from double burgers, double cheese, or double anything. Skip the bacon, large fries, and super-sized beverages. They can offer large-sized problems. Stick with regular or even child-sized portions.

Look for baked or broiled chicken sandwiches, even vegetarian burgers. Add lettuce, tomatoes, and pickles on a whole-grain bun, without mayonnaise. Try a sub sandwich once in a while. Sliced turkey or roast beef with shredded lettuce and tomatoes are good choices.

Limit any food that may be oily or creamy, or salads like tuna or chicken full of mayonnaise. These may sound healthy, but the extra oil and mayonnaise added to them makes them very high in fat.

Keep baked potatoes plain. When you add toppings, your potato can become laden with a lot of extra fat and calories. Top with fresh vegetables and maybe some lower-fat cheese.

Salads can be a good choice but not so good if you include higher-fat selections like cheese, croutons, and higher-fat dressings. Opt for many vegetables and top with a lower-fat dressing. Also beware of taco salads. These can be full of fat and calories. Fried taco shells, guacamole, sour cream, and refried beans can do wonders to adding up unnecessary calories and fat.

Always order your sauce on the side. It's best to add it yourself. Lemon juice, lower-fat salad dressings, and mustard offer better choices than higher-fat sauces and dressings. If you are going out for pizza, opt for the thin crust with vegetables, and, if you're daring, ask for lower-fat cheese. Pizza can be loaded with fat if it has stuffed crust, double cheese, sausage, pepperoni, or other high-fat meats.

Choose water, 100 percent fruit juice, or diet soft drinks over regular soft drinks, especially large-sized ones. Twelve ounces of a regular soft drink alone contains 10 teaspoons of sugar. How about those 30-ounce beverages, filled with 25 teaspoons of sugar, that everyone is drinking? *Wow!*

Fast food in the traditional sense is not your best choice. Many of the foods offered are higher in fat, calories, and sodium. These meals are notorious for being lower in fiber and vitamins A and C. If you order fast food, at least make smart selections.

Be careful with desserts, especially pies, cookies, and brownies. Choose an occasional small, low-fat frozen yogurt cone. These are tasty and not too fattening either.

Healthy Ordering—Made Easy

I'm all for diversity. I love it in our culture and in our foods. America truly is a melting pot with a lot of different flavors in our stew. We have a wonderful variety of ethnic eateries. There is even much experimenting at trendy restaurants where dishes are tastefully prepared with more than one ethnic flavor. The buzzword for this form of cooking is *fusion*. With all these culinary delights tempting our palate, let me share some helpful tips that can cut calories across the board-er!

WHAT YOU DON'T KNOW CAN MAKE YOU FAT	Adding butter, margarine, sour cream, creamed spinach, and extra cheese to baked potatoes can increase calories by as much as 200 to 500 calories per serving.

American Food Flare
American grills and family-style restaurants are available to consumers in many different price ranges. These restaurants typically cater to families who opt for a variety of food choices and selections. Healthier options include baked or grilled entrées, broth-based soups, and fruit platters. Veggies are always a plus. Avoid the cheese bread in favor of whole-grain bread.

Love Lasagna?
Italian meals can range from inexpensive to costly, from healthy choices to heavy, high-fat meals. Don't get thrown off by words like parmigiano, lasagna, alfredo, calamari, and cannoli. They may be Italian signatures, but the guidelines I've given you for a healthy diet still apply. Always ask how a dish is prepared before you order to be sure it is a smart choice. Beware of the extra oil and fat that are often used on appetizers and on pasta dishes. Many Italian restaurants now serve oil to pour on fresh bread. Use sparingly.

The large portions served at many Italian restaurants make them a perfect place to practice sharing. Healthier sauce options include primavera (not cream sauce), lemon juice, piccata (lemon-wine sauce), marinara (or tomato-based) sauce, red or white wine sauce, and light mushroom sauce. Artichoke hearts, sun-dried tomatoes, and garlic spices are healthy and yummy. Dessert can be guilt-free with a refreshing Italian ice.

Asian Food Feast

Whether it's Chinese, Japanese, or Thai, Asian restaurants are very popular. These foods are often considered healthier because of all the vegetables used in the cooking. This is where the unsuspecting consumer can be misled. Many of the entrées are extremely high in fat even if they come with veggies. For example, sweet-and-sour foods, tempuras, and fried entrées can kill a good diet. Don't worry! You still can satisfy your Asian food craving. Choose yummy steamed chicken, seafood, and vegetables. Vegetarians can feast on tofu (bean curd). Substitute chicken for high fat duck. Ask the server to hold the peanuts and crispy noodles and to reduce the oil. Find a restaurant that does not use MSG.

> ### Cyndi's Secrets™
>
> When you're sitting at the table, looking down on a half-eaten plate, ask yourself this question: Do you want leftovers to go to waste or to your waist? You decide. It's totally in your control—so share and take home a doggy bag.

Deli Dilemma?

Delis and sub sandwich shops are being advertised as healthier options to fast-food restaurants. Once again, buyer beware! Some foods here can fit that bill, but others do not. Portion sizes are often large, both in the size of the bun and the amount of meat piled on top. One good thing is that many sandwiches can be made to order. You can request healthier options including whole-grain breads, lettuce, tomatoes, pickles, mustard, and lots of vegetables. Choose sliced turkey, chicken, or ham. Be sure to leave off or at least limit the mayonnaise. Skip the chips. Have the server cut the sandwich in half and save for later. I have been known to order the kid pack. Free toy is optional!

Munching on Chips—Mexican

Mexican foods are delicious and flavorful. Ah, the spices and the salsa. I can hear the mariachis and see the margarita madness. Unfortunately, though, that tequila and high-fat sour cream are not good for your diet. You just have to be careful with your selections, particularly in fast-food Mexican-style restaurants. Salsa actually is a healthy option and so are fajitas, corn tortillas, burritos, and enchiladas. Just don't load your entrées up with heavy sauces, creams, or high-fat cheese. Eat your salad without the taco shell. For me, it's too tempting to eat the whole order of chips that are standard with most Mexican entrées so I have the server skip those. Nowadays, there are a slew of health conscious Mexican restaurants cropping up that serve fresh ingredients with no preservatives, lard, or MSG. Patronize these establishments. Olé!

Pizza, Pizza!

Most everybody wants a pizza on occasion. You can find almost any kind from the old classic thin crust with cheese to thick crust pizza stuffed with everything imaginable. Be careful with your pizza selections. Thin crust is the healthier option.

Load up the top with green and red peppers, mushrooms, onions, tomatoes, spinach, and any vegetable you can think of. Choose chicken or turkey sausage over high-fat Italian sausage or pepperoni. If you top it with cheese, request low fat. Start with a salad to fill up on greens.

Diet on the Go

Having a busy life is exciting and can be very fulfilling. However, it can kill your diet desires if you aren't careful. Whether you take your own food with you or eat out, choose to be a good dieter on the go.

Packing a lunch can offer many nutritious benefits that are certainly better than fast-food choices or the vending machine. When packing your own lunch, you know what goes into it and you can save money as well. A well-balanced lunch should contain a high-protein food, a starch, a fruit and/or vegetable, and a beverage.

Occasionally a treat could be thrown in too. Look back at the MyPyramid guidelines for healthy suggestions. Choose foods from each of the food groups. Limit excess snack foods, cookies, candies, and cakes that are high in fat and sugar. Select high-fiber foods like whole-grain breads, fresh fruits, and vegetable sticks.

Live YOUR *Life*

The best lunches consist of lots of variety. Keep the portions small and low in fat so that you become energized and don't feel like you have to take a nap!

Sandwiches are a common lunch choice. Seek out new fillings and breads to make your sandwich appealing. How about some sliced chicken or tuna? What about trying a sandwich wrap or raisin bread? You can even try a thermos of soup, cottage cheese, or yogurt. Packing a good lunch doesn't take a lot of time but it does take planning. If your mornings are rushed, then pack it the night before. Leftovers from home also make interesting lunches. When cleaning up, pack them into individual servings. Seek out containers that help keep foods fresh.

As a dieter on the go, you may choose to eat out. Make a conscious effort to plan and make wise food selections. As you become more knowledgeable as to what and how you should be eating, you will be able to eat out without a great deal of effort. Restaurants are finally trying to cater to consumers' requests. Many more choices are thankfully becoming available.

Sticking to a Meal Plan

Have you ever served a meal that just didn't look very appetizing? I've botched a few meals myself. I'm talking about that dinner of baked rubber chicken, mashed potatoes, and cauliflower on a white dinner plate that looked so boring and bland you fell asleep looking at it. How about that fresh stir-fry with a side salad that crunched when you chewed until you chipped a tooth? Meals like these often happen when you don't plan what will be served.

A meal should be appealing. If it is not, it will not be enjoyed. A proper meal should be one that is rich in the following characteristics: color, flavor, texture, and nutrients.

Cyndi's Secrets™

To easily plan your meals, do so on a cycle menu: Monday (chicken), Tuesday (fish), Wednesday (vegetarian), Thursday (beef), Friday (pasta), Saturday (leftovers), and Sunday (ethnic). Make a chart, and add side dishes.

Color

The color of your meal appeals to your eye and stimulates your appetite. Remember the meal described above—the all-white plate can be made more appealing by changing it to baked chicken with wild rice and fresh broccoli spears. Doesn't that sound better to you?

Flavor

Flavor is important, too! Spicy, sour, sweet, and tart are but a few of the many flavors available. All spicy or all sweet foods may be too much at one time. Try offering some mild beans or rice with a spicy enchilada, rather than a spicy side dish, to help balance your taste buds. The temperature of your meal should also be considered. Most people enjoy a balance of some hot foods with cold foods. Soup and fresh salad go well together, as does an omelet with fresh orange juice.

> **Cyndi's Secrets™**
>
> Color is an important things to look for in your diet. If you are eating a lot of colors, chances are you are eating healthy because of all the fruits and vegetables. Just don't eat too much food in gold like fries or brown like gravy.

Texture

Texture should also be thought out. People like the combination of soft foods with crunchy or chewy foods. Eating a meal should not require an excessive amount of chewing or no chewing at all.

Nutrients

A meal should be full of a wide range of nutrients. It is easier to put together a nutritious meal by choosing foods from the different food groups and planning a range of colorful food selections and various flavors and textures. Fiber is abundant in fresh, crunchy foods. Vitamins A and C can be found in both dark green leafy and red vegetables. Protein is abundant in meats, and calcium is found in dairy sources. Follow the MyPyramid guidelines and you can plan meals that provide your daily nutrients.

Shopping for the Goods

Nothing beats an old fashioned shopping list to help you plan for your healthy diet needs. Keep your list handy at home to help you and family members or roommates keep up-to-date on foods that need to be purchased.

If beer and ice cream show up more often than veggies and fruit you may want to start reading this book again. However, if you are finally trying to make healthy choices, the list can help you keep on target. Otherwise, impulse shopping can cause you to buy products you don't need. Consider MyPyramid and serving sizes—this will help you buy only the things you need, and in the right amounts.

Live YOUR *Life*

When time is limited, convenience items can be a good choice. Be wise when making your selections, and add complementary lower-fat side dishes to accompany higher-fat main dishes.

Prepackaged/Convenience Foods

Prepackaged and convenience foods are here to stay. Sure they can save time, but they also can run the food bill up rather quickly. Estimate the cost of preparing certain foods from scratch, and then compare them to the prepackaged item. See what the difference is for you? Making foods from scratch can also save you additional calories and fat. For example, making fried rice from a prepared rice mix is much more caloric than a quick, home-prepared version. If you are a fan of macaroni and cheese, you can use lower-fat cheese and milk when you prepare it yourself, an option that may not be available in a prepackaged type.

What about frozen dinners? There are entrées, family-size varieties, side dishes, and even special meals catering to children. Not all of these are good choices. Be selective. Choose the ones that offer standard serving sizes and use lower-fat preparation methods. You can even find them with vegetables and fruits that are often neglected in homemade meals. When selecting frozen meals, aim to meet these guidelines:

- Select meals with no more than 30 percent of total calories from fat.
- Select meals with no more than 200 milligrams of sodium per 100 calories.
- Select meals with at least 40 percent of the recommended dietary allowances for vitamins A and C.

Keep in mind that these guidelines don't guarantee that you will meet all your daily nutritional needs. In order to maintain a healthy intake, be sure to alternate your food choices. Try to limit everyday consumption of frozen meals. It helps to discover how to compensate for missing nutrients during other meals and snacks during the day.

Stocking Up on Staples

Having healthy choices readily available can help you lose weight. Begin by shopping at least once a week with a list in hand. This helps to ensure that you have a variety of perishable and lower-fat fresh foods to enjoy. It also allows you to have snacks and healthy meals around that won't kill your diet. There was a time when I personally hated to go to the grocery store. But then I discovered that my disdain was not for grocery shopping but because I didn't go enough.

When I finally would go to the store it was a big old long ordeal. Now that I go a couple times a week, I actually enjoy my visit. It feels like an old-world European escape to a foreign market where you have to shop daily for dinner. My kitchen is now stocked with lots of fresh fruits and vegetables. And even though I'm not the greatest cook in the world, I eat healthy daily. These days I'm all about "fresh," and I'm not talking flirty. That's another book, though. Anyway—let's dish on how to shop and stock those staples.

Learning the Layout of Your Supermarket

When you shop, try to do so at the same supermarket each week. Besides making friends with the butcher, baker, and cashier, get to know the layout and location of various foods. Supermarkets are designed to tempt you to buy more food than you need. Did you ever wonder why the milk and meat counters are always the farthest from the front door? Or why stores are now

Live YOUR *Life*

Shop the outer perimeter of your store for the freshest and most nutritious food choices.

baking bread in the afternoons? Milk and meat are the two most purchased items in the grocery store.

When you run in to grab a gallon of milk and end up walking up and down aisles, you can get tempted to pick up one or two additional items. Delicious baked breads smell so tempting when you shop at the store after work. Marketers plan this to appeal to you. How many times have you run into the store for one item and came out with ten?

One of my secrets is to shop the store's perimeter. This is where all the good stuff is—healthy fruits, vegetables, fresh meats, seafood, dairy products, and just-baked breads. The inside aisles mainly stock processed, convenience-type foods like canned goods, cereals, and cookies. Although you can't avoid the inner aisles altogether, knowing the layout of your store and a good shopping list can help you make the best food selections.

Guide to Stocking Your Home
Here are some healthy food options to stock in your home:

- Whole-grain breads
- Bagels
- Pita bread
- English muffins
- Rye or pumpernickel breads
- Raisin bread
- Sugar-free dry cereals
- Oatmeal
- Brown rice
- Couscous
- Bread crumbs
- Pasta
- Low-fat frozen waffles
- Skinless, boneless chicken breasts
- Lean ground beef or turkey
- Lean cuts of beef (flank, sirloin, tenderloin)
- Lean cuts of pork (canned, cured, boiled ham; Canadian bacon; pork tenderloin)
- Tuna, sardines, packed in water
- Fresh fish (white fish, turbot, fillet of sole, salmon), frozen fish without breading
- Skim or low-fat milk
- Eggs
- Low-fat cottage cheese or sliced cheese

- Low-fat ricotta cheese
- Nonfat or low-fat yogurts
- Nonfat or low-fat sour cream
- Parmesan cheese
- Low-fat granola or fruit bars
- Low-fat or fat-free cookies (vanilla wafers, gingersnaps)
- Fruit-filled cookie bars
- Low-fat crackers
- Baked tortilla chips
- Pretzels
- Popcorn (low-fat micro-wave popcorn)
- Rice cakes
- Apples
- Bananas
- Kiwi fruit
- Grapes
- Oranges/grapefruit
- Raspberries/blueberries/strawberries
- Pineapple
- Lemons
- Plums/nectarines
- Raisins/dried fruits
- Canned fruit (juice packed)
- Applesauce
- 100 percent fruit juices
- Carrots, baby carrots
- Celery
- Cucumbers
- Cabbage, napa cabbage
- Onions
- Broccoli
- Zucchini
- White or sweet potatoes
- Peppers (green, red, yellow)
- Lettuce, romaine, Bibb, spinach, or other varieties
- Tomatoes
- Frozen vegetables (without sauce)
- Canned tomatoes
- Tomato sauces, paste
- Canned beans
- Pasta sauces
- Pizza crusts
- Vegetarian burgers
- Low-fat soups
- Chicken/beef/vegetable broths
- Salsa
- Light mayonnaise
- Lemon juice
- Cooking sprays
- Balsamic/red wine vinegar
- Oils, vegetable and olive
- Mustard
- Light soy sauce
- Low-fat salad dressings

You do not need to purchase all these foods at once. However, having many of them around allows you to prepare quick and healthy meals without too much time or thought. Feel free to custom make the selections to include your personal favorites. Be sure to remove food that has been sitting in your home for extended lengths of time. Clean out items like candies, cookies, snack foods, and presweetened cereals. Begin to enjoy the fresh, delicious taste of wholesome, nutritious food instead.

Making Friends with Food Labels

This program can only work if you give careful consideration to what types of food you eat. It behooves you then to make friends with food labels. Nutrition facts labels found on food products inform you about the nutrients that are found in the items you buy. Food labeling guidelines are regulated by the U.S. Food and Drug Administration, while the U.S. Department of Agriculture governs the labels found on meat and poultry products. Federal laws require foods to carry nutrition facts labels on every product that is processed or packaged. The manufacturer's name and address, along with the food distribution company, must also appear, along with a nutrition panel that provides a listing of ingredients and standard nutrients.

Cyndi's Secrets™

If you haven't used a particular food in over a year, get rid of it. You will likely not use it (or want to use it) in the future.

Ingredient List

Federal law requires that all food ingredients be listed on the label. They have to be listed in descending order by weight and include all substances found in the food. This is important for people who need to avoid certain types of foods in their diet due to special dietary needs, religious reasons, or because of a food intolerance or allergy.

Health and Nutrient Claims

You have seen product labels that say "reduced fat," "low cholesterol," or "sugar free" to name a few. Some even claim to prevent osteoporosis or prevent certain types of cancer. Manufacturers deliberately place these claims on the packaging to help sell their products. In some cases these products may be a better choice, other times not. Once again, you have to be a savvy consumer. Just because a label indicates that the product is "light" doesn't always mean it is a lower in fat or calories; it could also be lighter in color or in sodium.

Thankfully, the federal government is regulating more of these claims. Health claims are based on scientific research showing evidence of the connection between foods or nutrients and specific diseases. Statements listed can indicate that a specific diet/health relationship exists, but statements cannot indicate that a certain food or food product prevents or causes a disease. Start comparing one product against another to determine which is best for you.

WHAT YOU DON'T KNOW CAN MAKE YOU FAT	Some food products are exempt from federal food labeling laws, such as foods prepared by small businesses, bakeries, and restaurants. Food in multiunit packages, those in small packages like chewing gum, and coffee and tea are also exempt.

The following health claims are the only ones currently permitted to be printed on food labels:

Calcium and osteoporosis: A calcium-rich diet is linked to a reduced risk of osteoporosis, a condition in which bones become soft or brittle.

Fat and cancer: A diet low in total fat is linked to a reduced risk of some cancers.

Saturated fat and cholesterol and heart disease: A diet low in saturated fat and cholesterol can help reduce the risk of heart disease.

Fiber-containing grain products, fruits, and vegetables, and cancer: A diet rich in high-fiber grain products, fruits, and vegetables can reduce the risk of some cancers.

Fruits, vegetables, and grain products that contain fiber and risk of heart disease: A diet rich in fruits, vegetables, and grain products that contain fiber can help reduce the risk for heart disease.

Sodium and high blood pressure (hypertension): A low-sodium diet may help reduce the risk of high blood pressure, which is a risk factor for heart attacks and strokes.

Fruits and vegetables and cancer: A low-fat diet rich in fruits and vegetables (foods that are low in fat and may contain dietary fiber, vitamin A, or vitamin C) is linked to a reduced risk of some cancers.

Folic acid and neural tube defects: Women who consume 0.4 milligram of folic acid per day reduce their risk of giving birth to a child affected with a neural tube defect.

Nutrient content claims are more specific than health claims. In order for a product to include any of these claims, the food product must meet appropriate criteria.

THIS CLAIM . . .	IS DEFINED AS . . .
Calorie free	fewer than 5 calories per serving
Low calorie	40 calories or fewer per serving
Reduced (fewer) calories	at least 25 percent fewer calories per serving than the regular version
Light or lite	a third fewer calories or 50 percent less fat or less sodium per serving than the regular version
Sugar free	fewer than 0.5 gram of sugar per serving
Reduced sugar or less sugar	at least 25 percent less sugar per serving
No added sugar	no sugars added during processing or packing, including ingredients that contain sugars, such as juice or dried fruit
Fat free	fewer than 0.5 gram of fat per serving
Low fat	3 grams or fewer of fat per serving
Reduced (less) fat	at least 25 percent less fat per serving
Lean (meats)	fewer than 10 grams of fat per serving, and 4.5 grams or fewer of saturated fat and 95 milligrams of cholesterol per serving
Extra lean (meats)	fewer than 5 grams of fat per serving and fewer than 2 grams of saturated fat and 95 milligrams of cholesterol per serving
Cholesterol free	fewer than 2 milligrams of cholesterol and 2 grams or fewer of saturated fat per serving
Low cholesterol	20 milligrams or fewer of cholesterol and 2 grams or fewer of saturated fat per serving
Reduced (less) cholesterol	at least 25 percent less cholesterol and 2 grams or fewer of saturated fat per serving
Sodium free	fewer than 5 milligrams of sodium per serving
Very low sodium	35 milligrams or fewer of sodium per serving
Low sodium	140 milligrams or fewer of sodium per serving
Reduced (less) sodium	at least 25 percent less sodium per serving

A Necessary Glance: Nutrition Food Labels

When purchasing a food product, take a look at the nutrition facts panel. Here you can find out what's in each serving you eat. The panel indicates the recommended serving size, number of calories in a serving, number of calories from fat in a serving, and amounts of nutrients per serving, including total fat, saturated fat, cholesterol, sodium, total carbohydrate, dietary fiber, sugars, and protein. Amounts for these nutrients are listed in grams or milligrams per serving as well as in percentage of daily values. Daily values are also required for vitamins A and C, calcium, and iron.

As illustrated by the table on the following page, the nutrition facts panel offers information to help you make good choices about the foods you eat. If you want to lose weight and modify caloric intake, it can help you purchase foods that help you limit your fat intake and total calories. The bottom of the nutrition facts panel offers reference information for you on daily intake limits of fat, saturated fat, cholesterol, and sodium, and appropriate intake for total carbohydrate and dietary fiber for both a 2,000- and 2,500-calorie diet. Most of us don't always remember these figures, so the panel is a great aid to help you see how a particular product fits into your total day's requirement.

Total fat recommendations are based on 30 percent of total calorie needs for the day. To determine your specific needs if you are not following a 2,000- or 2,500-calorie diet, you need to divide your total calories by 0.30 (30 percent). For example, if you are following a 1,500-calorie diet, no more than 450 daily calories should come from fat (1,500 x 0.30 = 450). To change this to grams of fat, you divide 450 by 9. (Fat provides 9 calories per gram of food.) Therefore, you should aim for a maximum of 50 grams of fat per day.

Nutrition Facts Panel

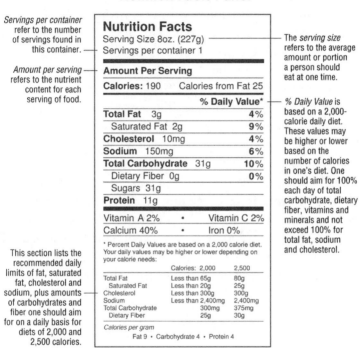

Servings per container refer to the number of servings found in this container.

Amount per serving refers to the nutrient content for each serving of food.

Nutrition Facts

Serving Size 8oz. (227g)
Servings per container 1

Amount Per Serving

Calories: 190	Calories from Fat 25

	% Daily Value*
Total Fat 3g	4%
Saturated Fat 2g	9%
Cholesterol 10mg	4%
Sodium 150mg	6%
Total Carbohydrate 31g	10%
Dietary Fiber 0g	0%
Sugars 31g	
Protein 11g	

Vitamin A 2%	•	Vitamin C 2%
Calcium 40%	•	Iron 0%

* Percent Daily Values are based on a 2,000 calorie diet. Your daily values may be higher or lower depending on your calorie needs:

	Calories: 2,000	2,500
Total Fat	Less than 65g	80g
Saturated Fat	Less than 20g	25g
Cholesterol	Less than 300mg	300mg
Sodium	Less than 2,400mg	2,400mg
Total Carbohydrate	300g	375g
Dietary Fiber	25g	30g

Calories per gram
Fat 9 • Carbohydrate 4 • Protein 4

The *serving size* refers to the average amount or portion a person should eat at one time.

% Daily Value is based on a 2,000-calorie daily diet. These values may be higher or lower based on the number of calories in one's diet. One should aim for 100% each day of total carbohydrate, dietary fiber, vitamins and minerals and not exceed 100% for total fat, sodium and cholesterol.

This section lists the recommended daily limits of fat, saturated fat, cholesterol and sodium, plus amounts of carbohydrates and fiber one should aim for on a daily basis for diets of 2,000 and 2,500 calories.

Keep the following tips in mind when reading food labels:

- Stick with listed serving size. Consuming more than this amount leads to higher calories consumed.
- Watch package sizes. Some products such as beverages, pre-packaged foods, and tuna may look like one serving, but

they are actually two. A trail mix I recently saw contained five servings even though it was packaged as a singular snack. Refer to the "servings per container" reference on the label for guidance.

- Look for high-fiber foods with at least 5 grams of dietary fiber per serving. These foods help fill you up and are often lower in fat and calories than others.
- Watch calories from fat. Make sure they're not your primary nutrient source.
- Balance your food choices. For every higher-fat product you choose, balance your meal with a lower-fat option. For example, balance cheese cubes with whole-wheat crackers.

In this chapter we talked about how you can eat well and still lose weight. It takes planning, shopping, reading, and understanding nutrition labels. All of these factors contribute to healthier eating habits and successful weight management. It doesn't happen overnight. Change takes time. Take it slow, and have fun as you morph into a healthier being for life.

10
Love Your Life and Results
Now and Forever

Obsession Stinks!

What good is getting great results if you aren't happy with yourself? Get over it! I can't tell you how many hot bodies I have met and or worked with who never seem to be satisfied. There's no nice way to say it: Body obsession stinks! It has a stench that has permeated Hollywood and now much of America. Being consumed with your weight is a formula for disaster.

First and foremost, get past the number on the scale. The number on the scale does not reflect on you as a person. Body weight fluctuates daily due to several reasons including water weight and monthly cycles in women. Focus on health, not weight. Think about how much better you feel when you eat well, lose weight, and love life. By putting all of those components together you can't help but look great, too—no matter what your size or shape. Loving life and your results now and forever is truly the sweet smell of success!

It helps to accept normal changes. Weight gain is inevitable as we age. Our metabolism decreases throughout our adult lives, somewhere in the area of 3 to 5 percent each decade. It's not unusual for men and women to put on an additional ten to fifteen pounds during their adult years. That amount of additional weight is manageable and should not pose major health risks. Now, if you have gained twenty or more pounds, you need to adjust your diet and lifestyle. The excess weight can become risky especially if it surrounds your body's vital organs. When this occurs, health risks including the risk of disease are increased and even premature death can occur.

Live YOUR *Life*

Losing weight and maintaining a healthy weight require much more than just cutting calories. They involve a lifelong approach to healthy eating and incorporation of positive lifestyle habits.

Accept yourself for who you are. Not everyone is tall or short. Nor is everyone thin and trim. If you have had a problem with weight your entire life, it may be difficult to make a total change to your body in adulthood. Just aim to be the best and healthiest person you can be.

Weight Loss—Your "Reality" Show

Reality shows are the TV hits of the day. Some of them actually offer some great advice while others suck. When I see the ones where people make major lifestyle changes in an hour, I wonder how long their new behavior really lasts once the camera is off. Well, since it seems like everyone on the planet has a program in production, why don't you star in your own "reality" show? The cool part is that you can make the results from your "reality" show last more than thirteen episodes. Your healthy reality can last a lifetime. Remember to set reasonable short- and long-term goals for yourself. Losing weight and being healthier and fit is important, but your goals should not get in the way of enjoying your life.

Some experts say that you should focus strictly on long-term health and forget about the immediate gratification of weight loss. Hey it's your show—your life! If trying to lose a few pounds within healthy limits before your class reunion or other major event in your life motivates you to live healthy, I say go for it! Just don't seek impossible targets that can set you up for failure. You can use the event as a kick start toward a healthy forever. That's an award-winning performance.

> **Cyndi's Secrets**™
>
> Body weight is not as important as body composition. The scale should not be your number one indicator of your health.

Make a commitment to stick to your goals. Constantly re-evaluate them. Use a weekly calendar or your personal dietary diary to jot down notes. Keep track of eating, exercise, and behavior patterns. Then note the changes you can make to your current habits. When you write them down, these goals become a constant reminder for you to follow. Take it one step and one day at a time. Soon enough, results will follow. Reward yourself (not with food, of course). Once you have mastered one goal, move on to another. This will keep you motivated over the long haul.

Staying the Course

Make gradual lifestyle changes. You didn't get where you are overnight, and you shouldn't expect to create new habits that quickly either. Making small changes will add up to big results. If it takes you months or a year to create new habits, work on them slowly. Each and every change can be beneficial in the long run. Don't worry! This doesn't mean you won't look good for a year. You can start looking and feeling better almost immediately. It just means you can keep getting better and better each day as you strive for your goals.

Live YOUR *Life*

There are no "good foods" and no "bad foods," only "good diets" and "bad diets."

We have discussed how you can have an effective weight-loss program by changing lifestyle habits. That means you need to eat healthy, exercise regularly, and maintain other healthy habits, such as avoiding smoking and limiting alcohol consumption. Habits that lead to problems with overweight and obesity now need to be replaced with habits that lead to health and fitness goals.

Small Changes Add Up

It may be easy to tell yourself to make all these changes. However, talking about them and doing them are two different things. A one-time overhaul is not the answer. It takes lots of small and practical steps to alter one's lifestyle. Take one day at a time. Initially you may want to try eating more slowly, or eating only at the kitchen table, to avoid grabbing second servings. Additional changes could include cutting back on an afternoon sugar fix snack twice a week, or not eating after 9:00 P.M., or even walking around the block once a day. Once you make a change and succeed, move on to another. Remember, small changes add up to big results. Do whatever works best for you.

Moving Past Plateaus

Anticipate ups and down. Gradual changes to your life-style will add changes to your overall weight. This can be really encouraging. However, your body has to adjust to changes and will unfortunately try to fight you along the way. You may initially lose some water weight, thus increasing your motivation to continue, but weight does stabilize and you will notice some plateaus. Be prepared for this reality. It is a very normal occurrence that has to take place for weight loss.

Plateaus are common occurrences in long-term weight reduction. You reach a point where the amount of weight loss levels off and the scale seems to read the same number no matter what you do. This is where most dieters get frustrated and give up. As you continue to lose weight, your body begins to adjust to its new weight. By doing so it becomes accustomed to meeting energy needs for a lesser weight. Losing weight becomes more and more difficult as you approach your weight goal. But it isn't impossible to get there. It just takes a little more effort. Don't view these plateaus as a failure but as a time to jump-start your plan. You can't avoid plateaus, but you can push through them successfully. Follow these tips to help you jump-start your weight-loss plan to the next level:

Redefine your goals: Address those areas that are most important to you now.

Evaluate your food intake: You may be consuming more than you realize.

Boost your exercise routine: Find ways to boost your metabolism; add an extra five to ten minutes each day, increase your intensity, and challenge yourself more.

Be consistent with keeping your diet and exercise diary: Keeping accurate records will keep you on track.

Accept Mistakes

We all make mistakes. Get past it and move on. Attempt to make better choices the next time. As you incorporate new changes into your lifestyle and aim to change your habits, you will slip back from time to time into old routines. Just become aware of these relapses. By evaluating yourself on a continual basis, redefining goals, and planning ahead, you can stay on top of your form. This helps you to get back up even stronger and happier in the long run.

Embracing Your Delicious Life

Once you achieve your weight goal, you are not finished. Weight maintenance becomes a necessity. Studies have demonstrated that a large percentage of people who lose weight actually gain it back within several months or up to a year after it is lost. Why? Simply stated, you can't go back to old habits once you reach your goals. That's why, with my program, I've tried to show you how to make your healthy lifestyle fun and realistic for you. I want you to love your healthy life and results now and forever. If you embrace these changes, you will truly stick with them because it is what you desire. Remember, this is a lifelong process, not a temporary change.

> **Cyndi's Secrets™**
>
> To avoid gaining your weight back, remember the key words—*balance, variety,* and *moderation*. In fact, don't just remember these words, live by them!

Once you reach your target weight goal, it is possible to eat more than before, but just a small amount more. To lose weight, I suggested you reduce your intake about 500 calories per day. To maintain, you can add those calories back, but not more. These additional calories don't go a long way, so don't get carried away with them. These should be added from each of the food groups, not just treats, and in balanced proportions.

Get to know your body so well that you are aware of any changes. There is nothing like what I call the "jeans squeeze" test. If you notice your clothes are beginning to tighten up a bit take immediate action. Cut back for a few days or a week to get back on track. It's a lot easier to lose one to two pounds than to take off ten or twenty. There is never an end to eating right and exercising regularly. No matter how old you are, embrace your delicious life.

Customizing Your Diet

Each and every day, new fads and trends crack into the world of dieting. Whether they are found in magazine articles, pills, powders, beverages, or equipment, more and more efforts are made to lure the public into quick weight loss. Some even come with good information and can yield positive results. What I find very alarming about most diet programs on the market, though, is that they don't allow for individual differences.

Let's face it, you are unique with your own set of health and life problems. You also have your own prefer-

Live YOUR *Life*

Engaging in a regular exercise routine, along with following a healthy, well-balanced diet, is the best way to maintain weight loss for life.

ences different from anyone else's. Is one cookie-cutter diet laden with rules and no flexibility really going to work for everybody? I don't think so. I love this program because it's flexible enough to take into account different health issues and lifestyle variances.

Cyndi's Secrets™

When you reduce food intake too much, your body will think you are trying to starve it. It will then protect itself by hanging on to all the fuel (food) it can get. As a result, your resting metabolism will decrease, thus making it more difficult to burn calories.

My program can even grow with you. As you get older, your dietary needs may change as your body does. I'm there for you. Now you have the tools to adjust to your many changing needs. For example, you can adjust your diet to make up for the lack of exercise in your life after a skiing accident left you with a broken leg. Simply re-calculate a new caloric goal and you are good to go. If you prefer to eat lots of little nutritious meals rather than three big ones, go for it. Maybe you like to do physical activity in ten-minute bouts rather than a single thirty-minute time slot. The choice is yours. There is a huge, wonderful range of healthy habits that are sure to fit your style and needs. You are free to customize and make this program your own!

It's a Brand New Day!

There's a widely used saying: "It ain't over 'til the fat lady sings." Well, this certainly isn't true with my program. For one thing, there are no fat ladies in my program, or fat guys, either. This diet requires that you think positive and visualize the new and improved you. I encourage you to quit thinking like a fat person. I'm not going to say think thin because thin is not necessarily better. However, you can think like the vital, beautiful person that you really are, no matter what your size. Celebrate your healthy transformation that starts right now, this very second. Follow the concrete plan of action that I have laid out in front of you. Keep reaching for your goals. Be sure to let me know how you are doing. Feel free to visit my Web site, *www.starglow.com*, and sign up for my *free* Cyndi's Secrets™ e-tips. Celebrate this fresh new start. It's a brand new day!

Yummy Recipes That Yield Results!

Recipes have been analyzed using the Food Processor II Nutrition Software. Nutrition information has been listed for total calories and grams of protein, carbohydrates, fat, and fiber per serving. (Optional ingredients and additional suggestions and substitutions are not included in the analysis.) Figures are rounded to the nearest value. Also provided are the dietary exchanges to help you determine to which food group each recipe contributes. All of this information is provided to help you determine the best options for your personal needs.

Vegetable Omelet

GETTING OFF TO A GOOD START

½ vegetable, 1 meat	
SERVES 2	
CALORIES PER SERVING 140	
PROTEIN 10 grams	
CARBOHYDRATES 5 grams	
FAT 9 grams	
FIBER 1 gram	

To save 50 calories and 5 grams of fat per serving, substitute 2 egg whites and 1 whole egg for the 3 eggs.

3 large eggs
2 tablespoons low-fat milk
Salt and pepper, to taste
1 teaspoon light margarine
1 scallion, finely chopped
¼ cup red pepper, finely chopped
¼ cup green pepper, finely chopped
1 teaspoon fresh parsley

1. In a medium bowl, beat together the eggs, milk, salt, and pepper.

2. Melt margarine in skillet over high heat. Add scallion and peppers. Sauté for 2 to 3 minutes, or until the vegetables begin to soften. Pour the egg mixture into the skillet over the vegetables. Cook for about 30 seconds, until the eggs begin to set. Use a metal spatula to lift the eggs, and tilt the pan to allow the uncooked eggs to flow to the edges. When the top portion of the eggs begins to set, fold the egg mixture in half to form the omelet. Transfer omelet to serving plate. Sprinkle with fresh parsley.

Blueberry Crumb Muffins

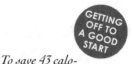

1 bread, ½ fruit, 2 fats	
YIELDS 1 dozen	
CALORIES PER SERVING 216	
PROTEIN 4 grams	
CARBOHYDRATES 35 grams	
FAT 7 grams	
FIBER 1 gram	

To save 43 calories and 2 grams of fat per serving, try the muffins without the topping.

¼ cup margarine, softened
⅔ cup sugar
2 eggs
½ cup low-fat milk
1 teaspoon vanilla
2 cups flour
2 teaspoons baking powder
Dash salt
1½ cups fresh blueberries, rinsed

Crumb Topping:
¼ cup sugar
¼ cup flour
1 teaspoon cinnamon
2 tablespoons margarine, softened

1. Preheat oven to 350°F. Spray a muffin tin pan with cooking spray.

2. Using an electric mixer, cream together the ¼ cup margarine and ⅔ cup sugar. Add eggs, milk, and vanilla. Carefully add the flour, baking powder, and salt to batter, combining until just mixed and moistened. Fold in the blueberries using a wooden spoon or rubber spatula. Pour batter into prepared pan to ⅓ of the way from the top.

3. Prepare crumb topping. In a small bowl combine the sugar, flour, and cinnamon. Add margarine and mix together using a pastry cutter or fork, until the mixture is crumbly. Sprinkle crumb topping over the tops of the batter.

4. Bake muffins for 20 to 25 minutes or until light brown and a toothpick inserted into the center of the muffins comes out clean. Cool before serving.

Yogurt-Peach Smoothie

1 fruit, 1 dairy, 1 fat
SERVES 2
CALORIES PER SERVING 186
PROTEIN 8 grams
CARBOHYDRATES 34 grams
FAT 3 grams
FIBER 1 gram

Try this smoothie with different types of frozen fruits, too—like blueberries, strawberries, and bananas.

1 (8-ounce) container low-fat vanilla yogurt
½ cup low-fat milk
½ cup frozen peach slices

Combine all ingredients in blender. Cover. Blend until smooth.

Orange-Banana Freeze

1½ fruit
SERVES 4
CALORIES 139
PROTEIN 4 grams
PROTEIN 4 grams
FAT 1 gram
FIBER 1 gram

This delicious frozen beverage will remind you of a Dreamsicle pop.

1 (6-ounce) can undiluted frozen orange juice concentrate
¾ cup water
1 (8-ounce) container low-fat vanilla yogurt
1 small banana, peeled and frozen

Combine all ingredients in blender. Cover. Blend until smooth.

Cranberry Bran Muffins

1 bread, ½ fruit	
YIELDS 1 dozen	
CALORIES 130	
PROTEIN 4 grams	
CARBOHYDRATES 28 grams	
FAT 1.5 grams	
FIBER 4 grams	

Try mini-muffin tins and make 3 dozen at 43 calories and 0.5 gram of fat per mini-muffin.

1 cup flour
1½ teaspoons baking powder
½ teaspoon baking soda
½ teaspoon cinnamon
¼ teaspoon nutmeg
2 cups (100 percent) all-bran cereal
1½ cups low-fat milk
⅓ cup brown sugar
1 egg, lightly beaten
½ cup applesauce
½ cup dried cranberries

1. Preheat oven to 375°F. Spray muffin tin with cooking spray.

2. In large bowl, combine flour, baking powder, baking soda, cinnamon, and nutmeg.

3. In another medium bowl, combine bran cereal, milk, and brown sugar. Set aside for several minutes. Add beaten egg, applesauce, and cranberries. Mix well.

4. Pour cereal mixture into flour mixture. Stir until just moistened; batter will be slightly lumpy. Do not over mix.

5. Pour batter into prepared muffin tin pan to ⅓ of the way from the top. Bake 20 minutes or until browned. A toothpick inserted into the center of the muffins should come out clean. Cool before serving.

Very Berry Smoothie

½ fruit, ½ dairy, ½ fat
SERVES 2
CALORIES PER SERVING 146
PROTEIN 8 grams
CARBOHYDRATES 23 grams
FAT 3 grams
FIBER 1 gram

Smoothies make a great choice for breakfasts on the go or for a satis-fying snack.

1 (8-ounce) container low-fat vanilla yogurt
½ cup low-fat milk
¼ cup frozen strawberries
¼ cup frozen blueberries

Combine ingredients in blender. Cover. Blend until smooth.

Grilled Cheese and Tomato Sandwich

2 breads, ½ vegetable, 1 dairy, 1 fat
SERVES 2
CALORIES PER SERVING 288
PROTEIN 13 grams
CARBOHYDRATES 27 grams
FAT 14 grams
FIBER 2 grams

Opt for low-fat cheese and reduce your calories by 57 and fat by 8 grams per serving.

2 teaspoons margarine
4 slices fresh sourdough bread
1 tomato, thinly sliced
2 slices Swiss or Muenster cheese

1. Spread margarine over one side of each bread slice. On unbuttered side, layer tomatoes and cheese. Top with other slice of bread, the buttered side out.

2. Heat large skillet. Place sandwiches in skillet. Cook for about 2 minutes on each side, until golden brown.

Spinach Crustless Quiche

LET'S DO LUNCH

½ vegetable, ½ meat, ½ fat
SERVES 6
CALORIES PER SERVING 81
PROTEIN 8 grams
CARBOHYDRATES 4 grams
FAT 4 grams
FIBER 1 gram

If you prefer, try a prepared crust, but beware of the extra 133 calories and 8 grams of fat you will add per serving.

2 eggs
2 egg whites
½ cup low-fat milk
1 (10-ounce) package frozen chopped spinach, thawed and drained
½ cup green onions, chopped
Salt and pepper, to taste
½ cup part-skim mozzarella cheese, shredded

1. Preheat oven to 375°F. Spray an 8" round quiche pan with cooking spray.

2. In large bowl, mix together the eggs, egg whites, and milk. Add the spinach, onions, and salt and pepper. Pour into prepared pan. Sprinkle with shredded cheese.

3. Bake 30 to 35 minutes or until quiche is light brown and cooked throughout. Cool slightly before serving.

Tomato Pesto Pizza

1 bread, ½ dairy, ½ fat
SERVES 8
CALORIES PER SERVING 154
PROTEIN 7 grams
CARBOHYDRATES 18 grams
FAT 5 grams
FIBER 1 gram

To jazz up your pizza and up the fiber, too, add fresh peppers (green and red), onions, mushrooms, broccoli, and any other favorite vegetables.

1 prepared pizza crust
2 tablespoons prepared pesto sauce
2 large tomatoes, finely chopped
2 garlic cloves, minced
1 cup part-skim mozzarella cheese, shredded

1. Preheat oven to 450°F.

2. Place pizza crust on baking sheet. Spread pesto sauce over the pizza crust. Top with chopped tomatoes, garlic, and mozzarella cheese. Bake 10 to 12 minutes or until cheese is melted and lightly browned on top.

Cheesy Tortilla Soup

1 vegetable, ½ fat
SERVES 4
CALORIES 75
PROTEIN 5 grams
CARBOHYDRATES 12 grams
FAT 2 grams
FIBER 2.5 grams

Try a cup with a half of sandwich for a quick (and light) lunch or dinner.

1 onion, diced
2 garlic cloves, minced
2 (14-ounce) cans vegetable or chicken broth
1 (14.5-ounce) can diced tomatoes
1 tablespoon chopped cilantro
1 teaspoon cumin
1 teaspoon chili powder
¼ cup low-fat Cheddar cheese, shredded
4–5 tortilla chips

1. In large saucepan, sauté onion and garlic in 1 to 2 tablespoons of the broth until tender. Add remaining broth, tomatoes, cilantro (if desired), cumin, and chili powder. Simmer for 20 minutes.

2. Strain and reserve liquid from soup. Purée remaining vegetables in blender. Return to strained soup. Mix well.

3. Pour soup into serving bowls. Top with cheese and tortilla chips to serve.

Cool Cucumber Salad

½ vegetable	
SERVES 6	
CALORIES 13	
PROTEIN 0	
CARBOHYDRATES 3 grams	
FAT 0	
FIBER 0	

This refreshing side dish makes a wonderful accompaniment to many chicken, fish, and beef dishes.

1 cucumber, peeled and thinly sliced
½ teaspoon dill
¼ teaspoon salt
¼ cup rice vinegar
1 tablespoon sugar
Dash pepper

1. Place cucumber slices in a medium bowl.

2. In a small bowl or jar, combine remaining ingredients. Mix well. Pour dressing over cucumbers. Toss well.

Easy Corn Chowder

1 bread, 1 vegetable, ½ dairy
SERVES 6
CALORIES PER SERVING 195
PROTEIN 9 grams
CARBOHYDRATES 36 grams
FAT 3 grams
FIBER 3 grams

You can cut down to skim milk and cut an additional 13 calories and 2 grams of fat per serving.

1 (14-ounce) can vegetable or chicken broth
2 (10-ounce) bags frozen corn (combine white and yellow, if desired)
1 small potato, peeled and cubed
1 onion, chopped
½ teaspoon salt
½ teaspoon pepper
3½ cups low-fat milk, divided
2 tablespoons cornstarch

1. In a large saucepan or Dutch oven, combine broth, corn, potato, onion, salt, and pepper. Heat to boiling. Reduce heat and simmer 15 to 20 minutes or until potato is softened. Stir in 3 cups milk.

2. In a small bowl, combine remaining ½ cup milk with cornstarch. Add to soup over low heat until soup thickens.

Orange Chicken

1 meat, ½ fruit, 1 fat
SERVES 4
CALORIES PER SERVING 234
PROTEIN 27 grams
CARBOHYDRATES 18 grams
FAT 6 grams
FIBER 0

Watch the size of the chicken breasts. Some are actually double the size of a 3-ounce portion.

1 tablespoon margarine
2 garlic cloves, minced
4 boneless, skinless chicken breasts
½ teaspoon dried rosemary
Salt and pepper, to taste
½ cup orange juice
¼ cup orange marmalade
1 teaspoon cornstarch

1. In large skillet, melt margarine over medium heat. Sauté garlic. Add chicken breasts, rosemary, and salt and pepper. Cook until chicken breasts begin to brown, about 3 to 4 minutes on each side. Remove chicken from skillet.

2. In a small bowl, combine orange juice, marmalade, cornstarch, and 3 tablespoons of water. Pour mixture into skillet. Heat 2 to 3 minutes, while stirring, until orange mixture begins to thicken. Add chicken back to skillet. Cover and simmer for 10 to 15 minutes.

Chicken Vegetable Stir-Fry

1 meat, 1 vegetable, ½ fat
SERVES 6
CALORIES PER SERVING 136
PROTEIN 14 grams
CARBOHYDRATES 6 grams
FAT 6 grams
FIBER 2 grams

Top with ½ cup chow mein noodles and add 20 calories and 1½ grams of fat per serving.

4 skinless, boneless chicken breasts
1 teaspoon salt
½ teaspoon pepper
1 teaspoon paprika
2 tablespoons flour
2 tablespoons oil, divided
½ cup chopped green onions
1 garlic clove, minced
1 cup fresh broccoli florets
1 red bell pepper, cut into strips
1 green bell pepper, cut into strips
½ cup chicken or vegetable broth

1. Cut chicken into ½-inch strips. In a shallow dish or pie pan, combine salt, pepper, paprika, and flour. Add chicken strips to flour mixture and coat well.

2. In a large skillet, heat 1 tablespoon of the oil. Add chicken. Cook until golden brown. Remove chicken to a large plate.

3. Heat remaining tablespoon of oil. Add onion, garlic, broccoli, and peppers. Cook until vegetables are slightly tender. Return chicken to pan and add broth. Cook until thoroughly heated and about half of the broth evaporates.

Lemon Fish Fillets with Capers

1½ meat, ½ bread, 1 fat	
SERVES 4	
CALORIES PER SERVING 206	
PROTEIN 19 grams	
CARBOHYDRATES 6 grams	
FAT 11 grams	
FIBER ½ gram	

Cook fish in 2 tablespoons of broth or use vegetable oil cooking spray instead of oil to save 60 calories and 7 grams of fat per serving.

¼ cup flour
½ teaspoon salt
½ teaspoon pepper
1 pound fish fillets (flounder, whitefish, fillet of sole, tilapia)
2 tablespoons oil
1 teaspoon margarine
1 tablespoon capers
1 tablespoon lemon juice or 1 fresh lemon

1. In a shallow dish or pie pan, combine flour, salt, and pepper. Add fish fillets to flour mixture and coat well.

2. In a large skillet, heat oil. Cook fish until lightly browned, about 3 to 5 minutes on each side. Remove fish to serving platter.

3. Remove skillet from heat. Add margarine, capers, and lemon juice to warm skillet. Heat until margarine is just melted. Pour sauce over fish fillets to serve.

Lentil Spaghetti

1 meat, 1½ bread, ½ vegetable, 1 fat	
SERVES 6	
CALORIES PER SERVING 315	
PROTEIN 16 grams	
CARBOHYDRATES 51 grams	
FAT 5 grams	
FIBER 12 grams	

Eliminate the feta cheese and reduce calories by 25 and fat by 2 grams per serving.

8 ounces spaghetti noodles
1 tablespoon oil
½ onion, chopped
2 garlic cloves, minced
1 cup dry lentils
½ teaspoon thyme
½ teaspoon salt
½ teaspoon red pepper flakes
1 tomato, diced
2 ounces feta cheese
2 teaspoons parsley

1. Prepare spaghetti according to package directions. Drain.

2. In a Dutch oven, heat oil. Add onion and garlic. Cook over medium heat for about 3 minutes. Add the lentils and 1½ cups of water. Bring to a boil. Add thyme, salt, red pepper flakes, and tomatoes. Bring to boil again. Reduce heat. Simmer, uncovered, for 30 minutes until lentils are softened.

3. To serve, place spaghetti onto serving platter. Top with lentils. Sprinkle with feta cheese and parsley.

Sesame Noodles with Peppers and Pine Nuts

2 bread, ½ vegetable, 1 fat
SERVES 6
CALORIES PER SERVING 219
PROTEIN 7 grams
CARBOHYDRATES 37 grams
FAT 4 grams
FIBER 3 grams

This pasta dish will jazz up your baked chicken breast or fish fillet.

8 ounces spaghetti noodles
1 teaspoon vegetable oil
½ red bell pepper, thinly sliced
¼ cup green onions, thinly sliced
1 (14-ounce) can bean sprouts, drained
2 tablespoons fresh basil, chopped
1 tablespoons fresh cilantro, chopped
2 tablespoons pine nuts

Dressing:

¼ cup lime juice
3 tablespoons soy sauce
1 tablespoon brown sugar
1 tablespoon water

1 tablespoon sesame oil
1 teaspoon ground ginger
2 garlic cloves, minced
Dash red pepper flakes

1. Prepare spaghetti noodles according to package directions. Drain.

2. In a large skillet, heat the vegetable oil. Add red bell pepper and onion. Sauté until slightly tender. Add drained bean sprouts and spaghetti noodles. Remove from heat. Toss with basil, cilantro, and pine nuts.

3. Combine dressing ingredients. Mix well. Pour spaghetti mixture into a large bowl. Toss with dressing. Serve slightly warm or cold.

Cinnamon Apple Chips

½ fruit	
SERVES 4	
CALORIES PER SERVING 54	
PROTEIN 0	
CARBOHYDRATES 15 grams	
FAT 0	
FIBER 3 grams	

*Make a bunch.
These go fast.
Just watch how
many you eat.*

2 apples, sliced very thin
1 tablespoon sugar
1 teaspoon cinnamon

1. Preheat oven to 200°F.

2. Cover a cookie sheet with parchment paper. Lay out apple slices in a single layer over the parchment paper.

3. In a small bowl, combine the sugar and cinnamon. Sprinkle over apples.

4. Bake for 1½ hours until the apple slices dry out. Remove from pan and let cool.

Yogurt Parfait

1 fruit, ½ dairy, 1 fat
SERVES 2
CALORIES PER SERVING 224
PROTEIN 7 grams
CARBOHYDRATES 47 grams
FAT 2 grams
FIBER 3 grams

Eliminate the granola to cut 40 calories and 1 gram of fat per serving.

1 (8-ounce) carton low-fat vanilla yogurt
¼ cup fresh blueberries
¼ cup fresh raspberries
1 small banana, thinly sliced
¼ cup low-fat granola

In two parfait or tall glasses, layer yogurt and fruit as desired. Top off with granola. Serve immediately.

Watermelon Ice

1 fruit, ½ fat
SERVES 4
CALORIES PER SERVING 74
PROTEIN 1 gram
CARBOHYDRATES 17 grams
FAT 0
FIBER 1 gram

Stick to a serving size of this refreshing ice treat. It's so good, you may be tempted to eat more.

4 cups frozen watermelon chunks, seeds removed
2 tablespoons sugar
1 teaspoon lemon juice

Place all the ingredients in a blender. Purée until smooth. Serve immediately.

Frozen Yogurt Sandwich

1 bread, ½ fat	
SERVES 2	
CALORIES PER SERVING 85	
PROTEIN 2 grams	
CARBOHYDRATES 15 grams	
FAT 2 grams	
FIBER 0	

Experiment with different flavors of frozen yogurt or sherbet for low-fat dessert treats.

2 graham cracker rectangles, broken into squares
¼ cup low-fat frozen yogurt, any flavor, slightly softened

Lay graham cracker squares onto a flat surface. Top 2 squares with frozen yogurt. Place remaining squares on top to make a sandwich. Serve immediately or wrap in plastic wrap and freeze until ready to eat.

Toss It Up Trail Mix

1½ bread, ½ fat	
YIELDS 2 servings (4¼ cups each)	
CALORIES 175	
PROTEIN 4 grams	
CARBOHYDRATES 29 grams	
FAT 5 grams	
FIBER 2 grams	

A combination of many snack foods can make a favorite trail mix. Play around with dry cereals, dried fruits, crackers, and nuts.

2 cups toasted oat cereal
1 cup pretzel sticks
1 cup small oyster crackers
½ cup dry-roasted peanuts
½ cup sunflower seeds, shelled
½ cup raisins
½ cup semisweet chocolate chips

In a large bowl, combine all ingredients. Mix or shake well. Store in air-tight container.

Chocolate Chip Meringue Bites

1 extra (sugar)	
YIELDS	3 dozen
CALORIES	34
PROTEIN	0
CARBOHYDRATES	6 grams
FAT	1 gram
FIBER	0

*These bites are
sure to satisfy
any sweet tooth.*

2 large egg whites
½ teaspoon cream of tartar
¾ cup sugar
¾ cup mini semisweet or milk chocolate chips

1. Preheat oven to 200°F. Line a cookie sheet with parchment paper.

2. In medium mixing bowl, beat egg whites and cream of tartar with electric mixer until foamy. Slowly add sugar. Continue beating at high speed until stiff peaks form.

3. Use a wooden spoon or rubber spatula to fold the chocolate chips into the meringue.

4. Drop meringue by tablespoonfuls onto parchment paper.

5. Bake 1½ hours. Remove from oven. Cool before removing from cookie sheet. Store in an airtight container.

Other Resources

CONTACT INFORMATION

American Dietetic Association
216 West Jackson Boulevard
Chicago, IL 60606
Phone: 800-366-1655
Web site: *www.eatright.org*

International Food Information Council
1100 Connecticut Avenue NW, Suite 430
Washington, DC 20036
Phone: 202-296-6540
Web site: *www.ific.org*

Food and Nutrition Service
USDA
3101 Park Center Drive
Alexandria, VA 22302
Web site: *www.fns.usda.gov/fns*

Food and Drug Administration
200 C Street SW
Washington, DC 20204
Web site: *www.fda.gov*

Food Safety and Inspection Service
USDA
1400 Independence Avenue, SW
Room 2942S
Washington, DC 20250
Web site: *www.fsis.usda.gov*
Food Safety Information
Web site: *www.foodsafety.gov*

National Eating Disorders Association
603 Stewart Street, Suite 803
Seattle, WA 98101
Phone: 206-382-3587
Web site: *www.nationaleating disorders.org*

National Association of Anorexia Nervosa and Associated Disorders
P.O. Box 7
Highland Park, IL 60035
Phone: 847-831-3438
Web site: *www.anad.org*

Anorexia Nervosa and Related Eating Disorders (ANRED)
P.O. Box 5102
Eugene, OR 97405
Phone: 541-344-1144
Web site: *www.anred.com*

President's Council on Physical Fitness and Sports
Department W
200 Independence Avenue, SW
Room 738-H
Washington, DC 20201-0004
Phone: 202-690-9000
Web site: *www.fitness.gov*

American College of Sports Medicine
P.O. Box 1440
Indianapolis, IN 46206-1440
Phone: 317-637-9200
Web site: *www.acsm.org*

Weight-Control Information Network
1 WIN Way
Bethesda, MD 20892-3665
Phone: 202-828-1025 or
877-WIN-4627
Web site: *www.niddk.nih.gov/ health/nutrit/win.htm*

National Health Information Center
U.S. Department of Health and
    Human Services
P.O. Box 1133
Washington, DC 20013-1133
Web site: *www.healthfinder.gov*

National Heart, Lung, and Blood Institute Information Center
P.O. Box 30101
Bethesda, MD 20824-0105
Web site: *www.nhlbi.nih.gov*

HELPFUL WEB SITES

www.cyberdiet.com: Offers helpful information for weight-loss success, including eating right, exercising smart, and feeling good.

www.self.com: Offers tips and articles on staying fit, eating well, and being happy.

www.afaa.com: Official site of the Aerobics and Fitness Association of America that offers information for fitness professionals and exercise enthusiasts alike.

www.niddk.nih.gov: From the National Institute of Diabetes and Digestive and Kidney Disorders, offering health, weight-loss, and weight-control information, research, and educational materials.

www.caloriecontrol.org: Provides information on reducing overall fat and caloric intake and achieving and maintaining a healthy weight.

www.thedietchannel.com: Offers helpful tips on successful weight loss, analyzing diets, nutrition information, and more.

www.weightfocus.com: Shares a collection of articles, diet and health information, weight-loss strategies, and more to help users achieve success in weight reduction and exercise.

Meal Plans Guide

Creating Meal Plans for Weight Loss

In this book, I gave recommendations as to the number of servings from each food group that should be incorporated into a daily diet. Suggestions included both recommendations for maintaining health and those for losing weight. Here, we will focus on those plans specifically designed for losing weight. The following meal plans meet these recommendations. You can choose to follow our sample plans or begin to create some of your own personalized plans, based on the same pattern.

The following menu plans are based on the 1,500-calorie guidelines. If you prefer to follow those guidelines outlined in the 1,200- or 1,800-calorie levels, you will need to adjust your food groups servings accordingly. Keep in mind that these plans are provided to help with some ideas on how you can prepare and consume well-balanced, nutritious, lower-calorie meals. Balanced food choices incorporating a variety within each food group

> MyPyramid.gov is your one-stop source for information. Take another close look at the Web site, specifically the "Food Intake Patterns" section.

and in moderate portions remain the key to healthy, low-fat meals. In order to maintain specific calorie levels, foods need to be prepared without excess fat and consumed in moderate portions.

Using Meal Plans to Meet Your Needs

The following two-week collection of menu plans provides just a sampling of the types of meals you can prepare for yourself and your family. Each offers a wide variety of food choices, balances food groups, and includes foods in moderate proportions. Personalized meal plans including the caloric requirements for your own needs can be provided by a registered dietitian. Should you need assistance with finding a registered dietitian in your area, you can contact the American Dietetic Association hotline at 800-366-1655.

Day 1

BREAKFAST ½ cup apple juice, 2 slices French toast, 1 tablespoon light maple syrup, 1 cup low-fat milk

LUNCH Sub sandwich (1 ounce deli-sliced turkey, 1 ounce deli-sliced roast beef, 1 ounce deli-sliced cheese, 1 small bun, 2 lettuce/tomato slices, and 1 tablespoon light mayonnaise), 4 baby carrot sticks, 1 medium apple

SNACK ¾ cup low-fat vanilla yogurt, ¼ cup low-fat granola

DINNER 3 ounces veal chop, ½ cup mashed potatoes, 2 spears steamed broccoli, ½ cup applesauce

Day 2

BREAKFAST ½ cup orange juice, ¾ cup bran flakes with raisins, 1 cup low-fat milk

LUNCH Chicken salad on pita (consisting of 3 ounces chopped chicken, 1 tablespoon light mayonnaise, ¼ cup cut-up grapes, ¼ cup water chestnuts, 1 whole-wheat pita bread), one wedge of watermelon (2 inches by 4 inches)

SNACK 2 squares of graham crackers, 1 cup low-fat milk

DINNER 3 ounces poached fish fillets, Parmesan noodles (½ cup wide noodles, 1 teaspoon Parmesan cheese, 1 teaspoon light margarine), ½ cup steamed zucchini, 1 cup tossed salad with 1 tablespoon low-fat salad dressing, 1 dinner roll

Day 3

BREAKFAST ½ grapefruit, ½ whole-wheat English muffin with 1 teaspoon fruit spread, 1 cup low-fat milk

LUNCH Hamburger (3 ounces hamburger patty, 2 lettuce/tomato slices, 3 pickle slices, 1 bun), 1 ounce pretzel sticks, 1 peach

SNACK Creamsicle shake (½ cup orange sherbet, ½ cup low-fat vanilla frozen yogurt)

DINNER Chicken stir-fry (consisting of 3 ounces chicken strips, ¼ cup broccoli, ¼ cup red pepper slices, ⅛ cup mushrooms, ⅛ cup bamboo shoots, 2 teaspoons soy sauce), ½ cup steamed white rice, 1 fortune cookie

AN EXTRA SNACK ½ cup Bing cherries

Day 4

BREAKFAST ½ cup pineapple/grapefruit juice, 1 sesame bagel with 1 teaspoon light margarine and 1 teaspoon fruit spread

LUNCH ½ cup low-fat cottage cheese, tuna/pasta salad (3 ounces tuna, 2 tablespoons light mayonnaise, ½ cup pasta, 2 to 3 lettuce leaves, 5 or 6 cherry tomatoes, ½ cup red pepper slices), ¼ cantaloupe

SNACK 10 to 12 grapes

DINNER 3 ounces London broil, ½ cup brown rice, 4 asparagus spears, 1 breadstick, 1 teaspoon margarine

AN EXTRA SNACK 4 vanilla wafers, 1 cup low-fat milk

Day 5

BREAKFAST ½ cup cranberry juice, 2 scrambled eggs, 2 pieces whole-wheat toast with 1 teaspoon fruit spread, 1 cup low-fat milk

LUNCH 1 cup tomato soup, 1 cup spinach salad with ½ cup strawberry slices and 1 tablespoon poppy seed dressing, 1 hard roll

SNACK 1 cup carrot/cucumber slices, 2 tablespoons low-fat dip (peppercorn ranch)

DINNER 4 ounces grilled salmon, 1 baked potato with 1 teaspoon low-fat sour cream, ½ cup green beans almandine, 1 (2-inch) square of cornbread

AN EXTRA SNACK ½ cup low-fat frozen yogurt, 1 small tangerine

Day 6

BREAKFAST 1 orange, ¾ cup bran flakes, 1 cup low-fat milk

LUNCH 1 cup vegetarian bean chili, 5 crackers, 1 cup leafy green salad with 1 tablespoon low-fat dressing, 1 French roll with 1 teaspoon low-fat margarine

SNACK 1-inch slice angel food cake, ½ cup fresh raspberries, 1 cup low-fat milk

DINNER 1-inch slice ground turkey meat loaf, 1 medium ear of corn on the cob, ½ cup steamed pea pods, ½ cup fruit cocktail

Day 7

BREAKFAST ½ cup tomato juice, 1 low-fat multigrain bar, 1 cup low-fat milk

LUNCH Chicken/rice salad in tomato (2 ounces chopped chicken, 1 tablespoon light mayonnaise, ¼ cup cooked rice, ½ cup shredded zucchini/broccoli/carrots, 1 tomato), 2 small clementines

SNACK 5 mini or 1 large rice cake, 1 cup low-fat milk

DINNER 3 ounces sliced turkey, ½ cup stuffing with chopped celery, 1 tablespoon cranberry sauce, ½ cup French-cut green beans, 1 slice sourdough bread, 1 teaspoon light margarine

AN EXTRA SNACK 1 apple, 2 gingersnaps

Day 8

BREAKFAST ½ cup pineapple juice, 1 poached egg, 1 biscuit, 1 teaspoon light margarine, 1 teaspoon fruit spread, 1 cup low-fat milk

LUNCH Roast beef sandwich (2 ounces roast beef, 2 slices rye bread, 1 teaspoon mustard), marinated cucumbers (½ cup sliced cucumbers, 1 tablespoon low-fat Italian dressing), 1 ounce baked chips

SNACK 1 banana

DINNER Chicken tacos (3 ounces chopped chicken, ½ cup shredded lettuce, 2 tablespoons shredded low-fat Cheddar cheese, ¼ cup chopped tomatoes, 1 tablespoon salsa, 2 taco shells)

AN EXTRA SNACK ½ cup sliced strawberries with 1 teaspoon confectioners' sugar

Day 9

BREAKFAST ½ grapefruit, ½ cup cooked oatmeal, 1 cup low-fat milk

SNACK ½ bagel, 1 teaspoon fruit spread

LUNCH Stuffed baked potato (1 medium baked potato, ½ cup steamed broccoli, 1 tablespoon shredded cheese, 1 teaspoon light margarine), ½ cup fresh fruit salad

DINNER 3 ounces pork chops, ½ cup wild rice, ½ cup steamed peas and carrots, 1 cup tossed spinach salad with 1 tablespoon low-fat dressing, 1 dinner roll, 1 teaspoon low-fat margarine

SNACK Fruit smoothie (1 cup low-fat vanilla yogurt, ½ cup frozen banana and/or berries)

Day 10

BREAKFAST ½ cup orange juice, 1 blueberry muffin, 1 cup low-fat milk

LUNCH Asian chicken salad (1 cup chopped lettuce, ½ cup chopped chicken, 6 cherry tomatoes, ½ cucumber sliced, ½ cup crunchy noodles, 2 tablespoons Asian salad dressing), 1 sourdough roll

SNACK 1 medium nectarine

DINNER Baked fish (3 ounces fish fillet, 1 tablespoon bread crumb coating, 1 teaspoon light margarine, 1 teaspoon lemon juice), parsley potatoes (½ cup chopped red potatoes, 1 teaspoon light margarine, ½ teaspoon parsley), vegetable stir-fry medley (½ cup sliced green and red peppers, ¼ cup onions, ¼ cup broccoli)

AN EXTRA SNACK 1 cup low-fat yogurt

Day 11

BREAKFAST ½ cup white grape juice, 2 slices raisin bread, 1 teaspoon light margarine

LUNCH Cottage cheese/fruit platter (¾ cup low-fat cottage cheese, ½ cup cantaloupe cubes, ½ cup honeydew melon cubes, ½ cup watermelon cubes, ½ cup pineapple cubes, ¼ cup mango cubes), 1 hard roll with 1 teaspoon light margarine

DINNER Spaghetti with meat sauce (3 ounces cooked lean ground beef, ½ cup spaghetti sauce, ½ cup spaghetti noodles), Caesar salad (1 cup romaine lettuce, ¼ cup croutons, 1 tablespoon low-fat Caesar dressing), garlic bread (1 slice French bread, 1 teaspoon margarine, 1 teaspoon chopped garlic or garlic powder), ½ cup sliced peaches

Day 12

BREAKFAST ½ cup grape juice, 1 cup multigrain oat cereal, 1 cup low-fat milk

LUNCH Tuna melt (3 ounces tuna, 1 tablespoon light mayonnaise, 1 ounce mozzarella cheese, 1 English muffin), 4 to 5 baby carrots, ½ cup pineapple slices

SNACK 1 ounce pretzel sticks, 1 cup low-fat chocolate milk

DINNER 3 ounces roasted Cornish hen, 1 medium baked sweet potato, ½ cup steamed baby peas, ½ cup rainbow sherbet

AN EXTRA SNACK 2 cups air-popped popcorn, ½ cup orange juice

Day 13

BREAKFAST ½ cup fruit cocktail, 1 hardboiled egg, 1 slice whole-wheat toast with 1 teaspoon light margarine and 1 teaspoon fruit spread, 1 cup low-fat milk

LUNCH Pizza bread (½ French roll, 2 tablespoons pizza sauce, 2 ounces mozzarella cheese), 6 cherry tomatoes, ½ cucumber, sliced

SNACK 5 vanilla wafers, 1 cup low-fat milk

DINNER Chicken kabobs (3 ounces grilled chicken, ½ onion cut into wedges, ½ green pepper cut into wedges, ½ red pepper cut into wedges, 6 whole mushrooms), ½ cup steamed brown rice, 1 cup Bibb lettuce salad with 1 tablespoon low-fat dressing

AN EXTRA SNACK 1 medium pear or 1 tangerine

Day 14

BREAKFAST ½ cup grapefruit wedges, 1 bran muffin with 1 teaspoon margarine, 1 cup low-fat milk

LUNCH Vegetarian omelet (2 eggs, ¼ cup chopped tomatoes, ¼ cup mushrooms, ¼ cup zucchini), 1 whole-wheat bagel with 2 teaspoons light margarine, 1 cup low-fat milk

SNACK 1 medium apple

DINNER 3 ounces grilled salmon, ½ cup potato wedges, spinach/orange salad (1 cup spinach, ¼ cup mandarin orange sections, 1 tablespoon low-fat dressing), 1 dinner roll with 1 teaspoon light margarine

AN EXTRA SNACK 5 mini or 1 large rice cake

As you can see, if you plan ahead you will be better prepared to shop and cook to meet your needs. Not only does it help to plan main courses, but it's also a good idea for side dishes and snacks. Developing a weekly or biweekly cycle menu plan can assist you in making the right choices for you and your family.

Index